Reconstructive and Cosmetic Surgery SOURCEBOOK

Health Reference Series

First Edition

Reconstructive and Cosmetic Surgery SOURCEBOOK

Basic Consumer Health Information on Cosmetic and Reconstructive Plastic Surgery, Including Statistical Information about Different Surgical Procedures, Things to Consider Prior to Surgery, Plastic Surgery Techniques and Tools, Emotional and Psychological Considerations, and Procedure-Specific Information

Along with a Glossary of Terms and a Listing of Resources for Additional Help and Information

Edited by
M. Lisa Weatherford

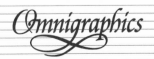

Omnigraphics

615 Griswold Street • Detroit, MI 48226

Bibliographic Note

Because this page cannot legibly accommodate all the copyright notices, the Bibliographic Note portion of the Preface constitutes an extension of the copyright notice.

Each new volume of the *Health Reference Series* is individually titled and called a "First Edition." Subsequent updates will carry sequential edition numbers. To help avoid confusion and to provide maximum flexibility in our ability to respond to informational needs, the practice of consecutively numbering each volume will be discontinued.

Edited by M. Lisa Weatherford

Health Reference Series

Karen Bellenir, *Series Editor*
Peter D. Dresser, *Managing Editor*
Maria Franklin, *Permissions Assistant*
Joan Margeson, *Research Associate*
Dawn Matthews, *Verification Assistant*
Jenifer Swanson, *Research Associate*

EdIndex, Services for Publishers, *Indexers*

Omnigraphics, Inc.

Matthew P. Barbour, *Vice President, Operations*
Laurie Lanzen Harris, *Vice President, Editorial Director*
Kevin Hayes, *Production Coordinator*
Thomas J. Murphy, *Vice President, Finance and Comptroller*
Peter E. Ruffner, *Senior Vice President*
Jane J. Steele, *Marketing Coordinator*

Frederick G. Ruffner, Jr., *Publisher*

Library of Congress Cataloging-in-Publication Data

Reconstructive and cosmetic surgery sourcebook : basic consumer health information on cosmetic and reconstructive plastic surgery, including statistical information about different surgical procedures, things to consider prior to surgery, plastic surgery techniques and tools, emotional and psychological considerations, and procedure-specific information; along with a glossary of terms and a listing of resources for additional help and information / edited by M. Lisa Weatherford.
    p.cm.-- (Health reference series)
  Includes bibliographical references and index.
  ISBN 0-7808-0214-4
  1. Surgery, Plastic. 2. Consumer education. I. Weatherford, M. Lisa. II. Health reference series (Unnumbered)

RD118 .R365 2001
617.9'5--dc21

                          00-066880

∞

This book is printed on acid-free paper meeting the ANSI Z39.48 Standard. The infinity symbol that appears above indicates that the paper in this book meets that standard.

Printed in the United States

Table of Contents

Part IV: Cosmetic Plastic Surgery

Part V: Additional Help and Information

Preface

About This Book

Derived from the Greek word "plastikos" which means "to mold or give form," modern-day plastic surgery offers a range of possibilities to all who seek to reshape, repair, or replace body parts. As a medical specialty, plastic surgery now benefits not only from expanded educational resources for surgeons, but also from the incredible advances of science in such areas as computer imaging and laser engineering. According to the most recent statistics from the American Society of Plastic and Reconstructive Surgeons, since 1992 the number of cosmetic surgery procedures has grown by 152 percent. In addition, reconstructive procedures comprised more than half of the 2.2 million plastic surgery procedures performed in 1998.

This *Sourcebook* offers general information about the practice of plastic surgery, what to expect, how to choose a surgeon, and how to know if a procedure is right for children, teens, and adults. More specific information also is provided concerning actual surgical procedures, surgical advances, and where to find additional information, help, and support.

How to Use This Book

This book is divided into parts and chapters. Parts focus on broad areas of interest. Chapters are devoted to single topics within a part. Some chapters are further divided into sections to provide additional detail.

Part I: Understanding Plastic Surgery provides an overview of the practice of plastic surgery, as well as the most recent statistics available concerning different cosmetic and reconstructive procedures and trends.

Part II: If You Are Considering Plastic Surgery addresses the decision making process including choosing a surgeon, psychological aspects such as motivations and expectations for teens and adults, and risks associated with certain procedures.

Part III: Plastic Surgery Techniques and Tools offers a look at some of the latest advances in plastic surgery from lasers to digital imaging to new skin grafting procedures.

Part IV: Cosmetic Plastic Surgery describes the most popular aesthetic procedures, how they are performed and what to expect before and after the operation.

Part V: Reconstructive Plastic Surgery offers a detailed overview of surgeries performed to repair birth defects and damage from illness and injury. These include procedures for the head and face, skin, transplantation and replantation, and gender reassignment.

Part VI: Additional Help and Information offers a glossary of terms often used in plastic surgery, as well as a comprehensive list of additional resources such as professional organizations, volunteer organizations, government agencies, insurance information, and support groups.

Bibliographic Note

This volume contains documents and excerpts from publications issued by the following U.S. government agency: U.S. Food and Drug Administration (FDA), Office of Consumer Affairs.

In addition, this volume contains copyrighted documents from the following organizations: American Academy of Facial Plastic and Reconstructive Surgery, American Cancer Society, American Society for Dermatologic Surgery, American Society of Plastic and Reconstructive Surgical Nurses, American Society of Plastic Surgeons, Facial Plastic and Cosmetic Surgical Center, Foundation for Reconstructive Plastic Surgery, Gender Reconstructive Surgery in Montreal, Massachusetts Institute of Technology, Plastic Surgery Network, Regions

Hospital—The Burn Center, Southern California Plastic Surgery Group, Mayo Health Information, The Voice Center of Eastern Virginia Medical School, and The World Craniofacial Foundation.

In addition, this volume contains copyrighted articles from *AORN Journal; Clinical Pediatrics; Insurance News Network, LLC; Medscape, Inc.; People Weekly; P/S/L Consulting Group, Inc.; The Canadian Journal of Plastic Surgery;* and *USA Today Magazine.*

Full citation information is provided on the first page of each chapter. Every effort has been made to secure all necessary rights to reprint the copyrighted material. If any omissions have been made, please contact Omnigraphics to make corrections for future editions.

Acknowledgements

In addition to the organizations listed above, special thanks are due to document engineer Bruce Bellenir, researchers Jenifer Swanson and Joan Margeson, verification assistant Dawn Matthews, and permissions specialist Maria Franklin.

Note from the Editor

This book is part of Omnigraphics' *Health Reference Series.* The series provides basic information about a broad range of medical concerns. It is not intended to serve as a tool for diagnosing illness, in prescribing treatments, or as a substitute for the physician/patient relationship. All persons concerned about medical symptoms or the possibility of disease are encouraged to seek professional care from an appropriate health care provider.

Our Advisory Board

The *Health Reference Series* is reviewed by an Advisory Board comprised of librarians from public, academic, and medical libraries. We would like to thank the following board members for providing guidance to the development of this series:

Dr. Lynda Baker,
Associate Professor of Library and Information Science,
Wayne State University, Detroit, MI

Nancy Bulgarelli,
William Beaumont Hospital Library,
Royal Oak, MI

Karen Imarasio,
Bloomfield Township Public Library,
Bloomfield Township, MI

Karen Morgan, Mardigian Library,
University of Michigan-Dearborn,
Dearborn, MI

Rosemary Orlando,
St. Clair Shores Public Library,
St. Clair Shores, MI

Health Reference Series *Update Policy*

The inaugural book in the *Health Reference Series* was the first edition of *Cancer Sourcebook* published in 1992. Since then, the *Series* has been enthusiastically received by librarians and in the medical community. In order to maintain the standard of providing high-quality health information for the lay person, the editorial staff at Omnigraphics felt it was necessary to implement a policy of updating volumes when warranted.

Medical researchers have been making tremendous strides, and it is the purpose of the *Health Reference Series* to stay current with the most recent advances. Each decision to update a volume will be made on an individual basis. Some of the considerations will include how much new information is available and the feedback we receive from people who use the books. If there is a topic you would like to see added to the update list, or an area of medical concern you feel has not been adequately addressed, please write to:

Editor
Health Reference Series
Omnigraphics, Inc.
615 Griswold Street
Detroit, MI 48226

The commitment to providing on-going coverage of important medical developments has also led to some format changes in the *Health Reference Series*. Each new volume on a topic is individually titled and called a "First Edition." Subsequent updates will carry sequential edition numbers. To help avoid confusion and to provide maximum flexibility in our ability to respond to informational needs, the practice of consecutively numbering each volume has been discontinued.

Part One

Understanding Plastic Surgery

Chapter 1

Plastic Surgery and Total Patient Care

This information is intended to assist those who have general questions about plastic surgery. It includes information about how plastic surgery fits into medical care, how plastic surgeons are trained, and the types of cases that plastic surgeons commonly treat. For more detailed information about a particular surgical procedure, contact the Plastic Surgery Information Service at 1-800-635-0635. Remember, each case is unique and a great deal depends upon the patient's individual circumstances. Specific questions about surgery can be best answered in a consultation with a board-certified plastic surgeon.

What Is Plastic Surgery?

Taken from the Greek word "plastikos," meaning to mold or give form, plastic surgery is the specialty of medicine dedicated to restoring and reshaping the human body. It encompasses both reconstructive surgery, which is performed on abnormal structures of the body caused by birth defects, developmental problems, injuries, infection, tumors, or disease; and cosmetic surgery, which is performed to reshape or restore normal structures of the body to improve appearance and self-esteem.[1]

History suggests that the practice of plastic surgery has ancient roots. However, plastic surgery as a defined specialty became fully

American Society of Plastic Surgeons, reprinted from The Plastic Surgery Information Service at www.plasticsurgery.org. © 1993; reprinted with permission.

recognized during World War I. Today, scientific advances in the field allow plastic surgeons to achieve improvements in form and function thought to be impossible 10 years ago.

Who Is a Plastic Surgeon?

A board-certified plastic surgeon is a doctor trained to be a concerned care-giver, a wound-care expert, a problem-solver, an artist-designer, and a meticulous surgeon in the operating room. It's important to realize that not every doctor who has claimed the title "plastic surgeon," has the same training. The truth is, anyone with a medical degree can call himself or herself a plastic surgeon; there are no laws that require doctors offering specialty care to meet certain qualifications.

In checking a plastic surgeon's credentials, patients are advised to consider a doctor who has completed an accredited residency training program specifically in plastic surgery. Such a program includes two or three years of intensive training that covers the full spectrum of reconstructive and cosmetic procedures.

Patients are encouraged to consider a doctor certified by the American Board of Plastic Surgery (ABPS). By choosing a plastic surgeon who is certified by the ABPS, a patient can be assured that the doctor has graduated from an accredited medical school and completed at least five years of additional residency training—usually three years of general surgery (or its equivalent) and two years of plastic surgery. To be certified by the ABPS, a doctor must also practice plastic surgery for two years and pass comprehensive written and oral exams.

Good credentials do not guarantee a successful outcome, but they can guide you to select a surgeon whose training and background will help you to meet your personal goals.

To Locate a Board-Certified Plastic Surgeon

Patients may call the Plastic Surgery Information Service at 1-800-635-0635 to receive the names of plastic surgeons in their area who are certified by the ABPS. This service, operated by the American Society of Plastic Surgeons, Inc. (ASPS), a national medical specialty society requiring ABPS certification as a condition for membership, can verify if a particular doctor is certified in plastic surgery, or has completed required training and is working toward certification.

Cases that Warrant a Plastic Surgeon's Care

Although much depends upon the patient's unique circumstances, there are certain situations that almost always warrant the specialized care that a plastic surgeon can provide. (See Problems Commonly Treated by Plastic Surgeons) Typically, a plastic surgeon is consulted when a child is born with a defect that affects function and/or normal appearance or when accident, injury, disease, or aging causes a physical abnormality. Plastic surgeons also are consulted in hand surgery, microsurgery, and craniofacial and maxillofacial surgery.

Emergency cases, such as facial lacerations, burns, trauma, and bite wounds, are also commonly treated by plastic surgeons. A patient who requests a plastic surgeon in the emergency room—rather than allowing the "on-duty" doctor to close a significant wound—is more likely to be satisfied with the end result.

Insurance Coverage

Reconstructive surgery is covered by most health insurance policies, although the specifics of coverage may vary greatly. Some carriers may fully cover reconstructive procedures, others may pay only a portion of the cost.

Cosmetic surgery, however, is usually not covered by health insurance because it is elective and not considered a medical necessity. Some plastic surgeons accept major credit cards or offer financing programs that allow patients to make manageable monthly payments for cosmetic surgery.

Keep in mind that there are a number of "gray areas" in plastic surgery that sometimes require special consideration by an insurance carrier. (See Procedures That May be Covered by Insurance) For example, eyelid surgery—a procedure normally performed to achieve cosmetic improvement—may be covered if drooping eyelids obscure a patient's vision. In assessing whether the procedure will be covered, the carrier often looks at the primary reason the procedure is being performed: is it for relief of symptoms or for aesthetic improvement?

The Other Doctors Involved

There are many cases in which a "team approach" is needed to best treat specific cases. Plastic surgeons commonly work in tandem with family practice physicians, general surgeons, pediatricians, oncologists, orthopedic surgeons, and neurosurgeons. Sometimes, numerous specialists are needed for a single case. For example, a child undergoing cleft-lip and palate repair might be overseen by a surgical team that includes a plastic surgeon, otolaryngologist, pedodontist, orthodontist, and speech pathologist.

A Consultation

A personal consultation with a plastic surgeon allows a patient to find out if he or she feels comfortable with the surgeon and his or her office staff. Typically, a consultation may take anywhere from 15 minutes to an hour. Some plastic surgeons offer no-cost consultations, while others may charge.

During the consultation, the surgeon will explain the procedure, the risks involved, and the probability of success. Patients are encouraged to bring a list of their own questions, as well as a note pad to jot down any information not included in take-home reading materials the surgeon may provide. The plastic surgeon will review a patient's medical history to evaluate any medical condition that might affect the surgical result. The patient's expectations and goals are also discussed, to make certain the desired surgical outcome is realistic.

Predicting Surgical Results

A patient's age, skin type, general health, genetic background, and the nature of his or her condition can all affect any final result. Patients who smoke may not heal as quickly as non-smoking patients. Patients with sun-damaged skin may not achieve the same degree of improvement as those without sun-damaged skin.

Though there is no way to exactly predict a surgical outcome, the surgeon will examine the known patient variables before surgery begins and can project an estimate of the surgical result. Patients can take comfort in knowing that most of the procedures performed today have been refined over several decades.

In recent years, some plastic surgeons have begun using computer-imaging machines during consultations to show patients an estimate of post-operative appearance. A photograph of the patient is transferred to a computer screen and then altered by the surgeon to approximate the post-operative result. Doctors who use imaging find that computer-generated pictures can enhance doctor-patient communication. It's important for the patient to realize that a computer image may not match reality and represents no guarantee of outcome.

No computer can take into account a patient's skin elasticity, bone structure, blood supply, and healing ability.

Types of Anesthesia Used by Plastic Surgeons

Three basic types of anesthesia are used for plastic surgery procedures. A local injection, which numbs only the immediate area to be operated on, is used mainly for less invasive procedures. Local injection plus sedation allows the patient to remain awake, yet relaxed through the entire procedure and is a common type of anesthesia used for cosmetic surgery procedures. General anesthesia, which allows a patient to sleep though the procedure, is usually used when large areas of the body are involved, or in children.

Where Are Most Plastic Surgery Procedures Performed?

Whether a procedure is performed in an in-office surgical facility, a hospital, or a freestanding surgery center usually depends upon the complexity of the operation and the plastic surgeon's recommendation.

For cost-containment and convenience, an increasing number of procedures—especially cosmetic operations—are being performed in freestanding or office-based surgical facilities on an outpatient basis. Patients planning to have surgery in this type of facility should ensure that it is properly equipped and staffed, that it has access to a nearby hospital, that the anesthesia will be administered by a well-trained professional, and that the doctor has privileges to perform the same procedure at an accredited hospital.

One additional sign of a quality facility is accreditation by the American Association for Accreditation of Ambulatory Plastic Surgery Facilities (AAAAPSF). This organization not only inspects the facility itself, it requires that the practicing physicians are certified in plastic surgery and have operating privileges at a local accredited hospital. AAAAPSF re-inspects facilities every three years. A patient can check if a plastic surgeon's facility is accredited by phoning ASPS at 1-800-635-0635.

Problems Commonly Treated by Plastic Surgeons[2]

Birth Defects and Developmental Abnormalities

- Birthmarks, including port-wine stains and hemangiomas, congenital nevi

- Abnormal breast development
- Cleft-lip and palate deformities
- Hand deformities
- Skull and facial bone deformities
- Prominent and deformed ears

Acquired Deformities Including those Resulting from Trauma or Disease

- Scars
- Wounds, soft tissue deformity from trauma or disease
- Burn scars
- Growths and tissue defects including cancer treatment and mastectomy
- Poorly healed wounds, scars that limit movement
- Lacerations
- Severed limbs, fingers or toes
- Skull and jaw injuries
- Drooping brow and upper eyelids, which impair vision
- Hand injuries and acquired problems
- Congenital and developmental breast deformity

Cosmetic Concerns

- Excess body fat
- Disproportionate or sagging breasts
- Skin problems: wrinkling, uneven pigmentation, sun damage, unwanted tattoos
- Sagging facial skin and muscles, loose neck skin
- Hair loss
- Facial features to improve the appearance of the nose, cheekbones, chin shapes

* This is a partial list.

Procedures That May be Covered by Insurance [3]

Abdominal Surgery, When It Is Performed to:

- alleviate health problems, such as back pain, sores, rashes, hernia;
- restore the ability to walk normally.

Breast Surgery, When It Is Performed to:

- correct congenital asymmetry;
- reduce overly-large breasts that are causing health problems (shoulder grooving, neck and back pain, etc.);
- reconstruct a breast lost to disease;
- correct congenital absence of breast;
- reduce over-developed male breasts—gynecomastia.

Ear Surgery, When It Is Performed to:

- correct congenitally-deformed ears;
- reconstruct ears that are deformed by disease or injury.

Eyelid Surgery, When It Is Performed to:

- correct drooping upper eyelids that are obscuring vision;
- correct out-turned or in-turned lower eyelids.

Facial Surgery, When It Is Performed to:

- correct an asymmetrical appearance caused by facial paralysis;
- treat conditions affecting the facial muscles, lips, and cheeks;
- treat traumatic deformities;
- correct head and neck deformities.

Hand Surgery, When It Is Performed to:

- treat carpal tunnel syndrome;
- correct Dupuytren's contracture, treat tendon and nerve injuries;
- correct syndactyly (fused fingers) and other congenital deformities.

Nasal Surgery, When It Is Performed to:

- correct deformities resulting from birth defects or disease;
- treat injuries or nasal deformities that may affect breathing.

For More Information

Additional statistical information on plastic surgery is available from the Plastic Surgery Information Service web site at www.plastic surgery.org or call (800) 635-0635.

Notes

[1]Definition as adopted by the American Medical Association (AMA) and the American Society of Plastic Surgeons (ASPS).

[2]Numerous individual circumstances affect whether a procedure is covered. Patients should obtain written verification of coverage and prior authorization for the treatment from their carriers.

[3] Ibid.

Chapter 2

Plastic Surgery Statistics

About the Tables in This Chapter

The following information is from the American Society of Plastic Surgeons' (ASPS) National Clearinghouse of Plastic Surgery Statistics. The ASPS represents more than 5,000 plastic surgeons certified by the American Board of Plastic Surgery and is the leading authority on plastic surgery. This information is compiled by the ASPS as part of its comprehensive overview of plastic surgery performed in the United States. Additional statistical information on plastic surgery is available from the Plastic Surgery Information Service web site at www.plasticsurgery.org or call (800) 635-0635.

This chapter presents the following tables:

- **Table 2.1.** Age Distribution: Cosmetic Procedures
- **Table 2.2.** Reconstructive Procedure Trends
- **Table 2.3.** Cosmetic Surgery Trends
- **Table 2.4.** Fee Structures: Average Surgeons' Fees

Note: Please credit the American Society of Plastic Surgeons (ASPS) when citing statistical data.

American Society of Plastic Surgeons, reprinted from the Plastic Surgery Information Service at http://www.plasticsurgery.org. © 1998; reprinted with permission.

Table 2.1. 1998 Age Distribution: Cosmetic Procedures

(Percentages indicate percent of national cosmetic total. Top five procedures indicated in bold.) ASPS Procedural Statistics represent procedures performed by 97 percent of all physicians certified by the American Board of Plastic Surgery.

Procedure Name	18 or less		19-34		35-50		51-64		65+	
Breast augmentation	**1,840**	1%	**79,341**	60%	**46,380**	35%	3,486	3%	1,330	1%
Breast implant removal	N/A		N/A		N/A		N/A		N/A	
Breast lift	406	1%	10,036	32%	15,766	50%	4,508	14%	809	3%
Breast reduction in men	**1,862**	21%	4,121	46%	1,967	22%	783	9%	291	3%
Buttock lift	0		251	20%	752	60%	243	19%	0	
Cheek implants	36	1%	555	19%	1,437	50%	629	22%	207	7%
Chemical peel	491	1%	**10,702**	16%	**31,452**	48%	**15,819**	24%	**7,538**	11%
Chin augmentation	204	4%	1,402	29%	1,869	39%	1,060	22%	259	5%
Collagen injection	298	1%	5,516	12%	21,159	46%	14,397	31%	4,480	10%
Dermabrasion	1,317	11%	2,325	19%	2,996	25%	4,720	39%	833	7%
Ear surgery **	**4,721**	59%	1,941	24%	1,406	17%	N/A		N/A	
Eyelid surgery	126	*	4,052	3%	**41,109**	34%	**45,306**	38%	**29,408**	25%
Facelift	34	*	360	1%	18,457	26%	**38,792**	55%	**13,304**	19%
Fat injections	244	1%	4,027	16%	10,534	41%	8,738	34%	1,894	8%
Forehead lift	0		803	2%	14,963	41%	16,487	45%	4,523	12%
Laser skin resurfacing	1,005	2%	5,963	11%	22,932	41%	19,330	35%	6,393	11%
Liposuction	1,645	1%	**46,745**	27%	**86,400**	50%	**29,499**	17%	**7,790**	5%

Table 2.1. 1998 Age Distribution: Cosmetic Procedures, continued

Procedure Name	18 or less		19-34		35-50		51-64		65+	
Male-pattern baldness	0		391	18%	1,512	70%	244	11%	0	
Nose reshaping	8,074	14%	25,494	46%	15,717	28%	4,894	9%	1,774	3%
Retin-A treatment	2,224	2%	23,313	22%	51,756	48%	22,016	21%	7,553	7%
Thigh lift	19	1%	650	17%	2,254	60%	776	21%	86	2%
Tummy tuck	56	*	9,833	21%	25,472	55%	9,351	20%	1,886	4%
Upper arm lift	19	1%	269	14%	924	48%	615	32%	111	6%
Wrinkle injection (fibril)	2	*	5	*	280	19%	734	50%	442	30%
Totals+	**24,623**	**2%**	**238,095**	**23%**	**417,494**	**41%**	**242,427**	**24%**	**90,911**	**9%**

+All figures are projected. Figures and percentages may not add to 100% due to rounding.
*Denotes less than 1%.
**Following are further age breakdowns for ear surgery:

6 or less	970
7-12	1,968
13-18	1,783

35-50 year old total represents all patients 35 and older.

13

Table 2.2. Reconstructive Procedures—Trends: 1992, 1996, 1997, 1998

	Total	Total	Total	Total	Percent Change	Percent Change
	1992[1]	1996	1997	1998	1992 vs. 1998	1996 vs. 1998
Birth Defects	33,501	29,214	34,587	22,457	-33%	-23%
Breast Reconstruction	29,607	42,454	50,337	69,683	135%	64%
Breast Reduction	39,639	57,679	64,620	70,358	77%	22%
Burn Care	17,552	25,177		27,875	59%	11%
Animal Bites	10,376	12,366		10,152	-2%	-18%
Hand	138,233	153,581	137,040	160,671	16%	5%
Lacerations	135,494	115,998	104,584	72,818	-46%	-37%
Maxillofacial	22,095	28,338		22,516	2%	-21%
Microsurgical (other than breast)	19,405	21,337		24,573	27%	15%
Scar Revision	52,647	50,952		47,100	-11%	-8%
Subcutaneous Mastectomy	2,458	1,766		1,500	-39%	-15%
Tumor Removal	502,567	542,063	563,059	509,457	1%	-6%
Breast Implant Removals (Reconstructive Patients)	7,379	11,366		11,419	55%	0%
All other reconstructive procedures	116,737	146,470		116,620	0%	-20%

Table 2.2. Reconstructive Procedures—Trends: 1992, 1996, 1997, 1998, continued.

	Total 1992¹	Total 1996	Total 1997	Total 1998	Percent Change 1992 vs. 1998	Percent Change 1996 vs. 1998
All other reconstructive endoscopic	N/A	2,214		2,235	N/A	1%
Total Reconstructive	1,127,890	1,240,973		1,169,434	4%	-6%
Total Reconstructive (6 procedures reported in 1997)			954,227			

Additional information on plastic surgery is available from the Plastic Surgery Information Service web site at www.plasticsurgery.org or call (800) 635-0635.

¹The 1992 Procedural Statistics have been adjusted to incorporate breast implant removals for purposes of comparison with 1996 statistics, when the procedure was incorporated as a part of the total.

15

Table 2.3. Cosmetic Surgery Trends: 1992, 1996, 1997, 1998

Top five procedures indicated in bold.

	Total 1992	Total 1996	Total 1997+	Total 1998	% Change 1992 vs. 1998	% Change 1996 vs. 1998
Breast augmentation	32,607	**87,704**	**122,285**	**132,378**	**306%**	51%
Breast implant removal	18,297	3,013	N/A	32,262**	76%	**971%****
Breast lift	7,963	16,097	N/A	31,525	296%	**96%**
Breast reduction in men	4,997	6,045	N/A	9,023	81%	49%
Buttock lift	291*	774*	N/A	1,246	**328%**	61%
Buttock implant	15	N/A	N/A	N/A	N/A	N/A
Calf implant	196	N/A	N/A	N/A	N/A	N/A
Cheek implants	1,741	2,257	N/A	2,864	65%	27%
Chemical Peel	19,049	42,628	N/A	66,002	246%	55%
Chin augmentation	4,115	4,797	N/A	4,795	17%	0%
Collagen injections	**41,623**	34,091	N/A	45,851	10%	34%
Dermabrasion	13,457	7,975	N/A	12,191	-9%	53%
Ear surgery	6,371	7,192	N/A	8,069	27%	12%
Eyelid surgery	**59,461**	**76,242**	**110,709**	**120,001**	102%	57%
Facelift	**40,077**	**53,435**	**61,692**	**70,947**	77%	33%
Fat injections	7,865	13,654	N/A	25,437	223%	**86%**

Table 2.3. Cosmetic Surgery Trends: 1992, 1996, 1997, 1998, continued.

Total	Total 1992	Total 1996	Total 1997+	Total 1998	% Change 1992 vs. 1998	% Change 1996 vs. 1998
Forehead lift	13,501	22,864	N/A	36,777	172%	61%
Laser skin resurfacing	N/A	46,263	36,860	55,623	N/A	20%
Liposuction	**47,212**	**109,353**	**149,042**	**172,079**	264%	57%
Male-pattern baldness	1,955	4,042	N/A	2,146	10%	-47%
Nose reshaping	**50,175**	45,977	**48,620**	55,953	12%	22%
Pectoral implant	96	N/A	N/A	N/A	N/A	N/A
Retin-A treatment	23,520	**74,382**	N/A	**106,862**	**354%**	44%
Thigh lift	1,023	2,114	N/A	3,785	270%	**79%**
Tummy tuck	16,810	34,235	N/A	46,597	177%	36%
Upper arm lift	434*	1,614	N/A	1,939	**347%**	20%
Wrinkle injection (fibril)	357*	164	N/A	1,463	310%	**792%**
Total	**413,208***	**696,904**	**529,208+**	**1,045,815**	**153%**	**50%**

+Only six procedures tracked in 1997

**83 percent of implants were replaced.

*Caution: small sample sizes.

***The Total is lower for 1992 because Laser Skin Resurfacing was not reported in that year.

17

Table 2.4. 1998 Average Surgeons Fees: Cosmetic and Reconstructive Procedures

Procedural statistics represent procedures performed by 97 percent of all physicians certified by the American Board of Plastic Surgery.

Procedure	National Average[1]	
Breast augmentation	$3,077	($3,292)[2]
Breast lift	$3,426	
Breast reconstruction		
Implant alone	$2,971	
Tissue expander	$3,567	
Latissimus dorsi muscul. Flap	$5,468	
TRAM (pedicle) flap	$7,252	
Microsurgical free flap	$9,435	
Breast reduction	$5,471	
Breast reduction in men	$2,786	
Buttock lift	$3,693	
Cheek implants	$2,135	
Chemical peel		
Full face	$1,353	
Regional	$629	
Chin augmentation		
Implant	$1,583	
Osteotomy	$1,998	
Collagen injections—per 1cc injection	$315	
Dermabrasion	$1,578	
Ear surgery	$2,501	
Eyelid surgery		
Both uppers	$1,734	
Both lowers	$1,785	
Combination of both	$2,942	
Facelift	$4,991	($4,795)[2]
Fat injection		
Head/Neck	$1,093	
Trunk	$88	
Extremities	$917	
Forehead lift	$2,526	($2,649)[2]

Table 2.4. 1998 Average Surgeons Fees: Cosmetic and
Reconstructive Procedures, continued.

Procedural statistics represent procedures performed by 97 percent of all physicians certified by the American Board of Plastic Surgery.

Procedure	National Average[1]	
Laser skin resurfacing		
Full face	$2,770	
Partial face	$1,296	
Liposuction—any single site	$1,872	
Ultrasound assisted liposuction—any single site	$3,817	
Male-pattern baldness		
Scalp reduction—all stages	$2,776	
Pedicle flap—all stages	$3,942	
Tissue expansion—all stages	$4,233	
Nose reshaping (primary)		
Fee for open rhinoplasty	$3,434	
Fee for closed rhinoplasty	$3,023	
Nose reshaping (secondary)		
Fee for open rhinoplasty	$3,304	
Fee for closed rhinoplasty	$2,928	
Retin-A® treatment—per visit	$82	
Thigh lift	$3,817	
Tummy tuck	$4,095	($4,326)[2]
Upper arm lift	$2,820	
Wrinkle injection (fibril)	$390	

[1] Fees generally vary according to region of country and patient needs. These
fees are averages only. In general, fees do not include anesthesia, operating room
facilities or other related expenses.

[2] Averages for procedure that are being performed specifically with an endoscope
are reported in parentheses.

Note: Please credit the American Society of Plastic Surgeons (ASPS) when citing statistical data.

Part Two

If You Are Considering Plastic Surgery

Chapter 3

How to Choose a Plastic Surgeon

Selecting the surgeon has to be the single most important factor in the success of your plastic surgery. Here are some tips to keep in mind when selecting your plastic surgeon. Remember, all the surgeons listed with "Plastic Surgery Network" are Board Certified.

Be sure that the plastic surgeon you choose has the following qualifications:

1. Certification by the American Board of Plastic Surgery, or the American Board of Facial Plastic Surgery: Such certification means that the surgeon has completed his/her training to be a plastic surgeon, or a facial plastic surgeon respectively, and also has passed the examinations given by the board.

2. Membership in the Plastic Surgery or Cosmetic Surgery Societies of their corresponding field of surgery or specialty.

3. Hospital affiliation: Although many plastic surgery procedures are performed in the office, always check with your surgeon about his/her hospital affiliation and that he/she has the privileges to perform the procedure of your interest in that hospital.

4. Initial consultation with your surgeon: Make an appointment for an initial consultation with the surgeon you chose. The

surgeon will be able to answer the rest of your questions, explain the procedure, its risks and potential complications for you. You should discuss with your surgeon your expectations, and any related matter that may affect your recovery like the nature of your job, smoking or drinking habits, other diseases or medications you are using, and any related personal matters.

5. References: Ask the plastic surgeon for references and a list of his/her patients. Call these references and talk to them. Ask to see some of the photographs of patients who underwent similar procedures.

For additional information and/or personal consultation, please find the plastic surgeon nearest you in our Plastic Surgeon Locator at http://www.plastic-surgery.net.

Have a successful surgery and post operative recovery.

Chapter 4

Psychological Aspects of Plastic Surgery

Improving Your Self-Image with Plastic Surgery

Each of us has a "self-image," a perception of how we believe we look to others. People who are happy with their self-image are more likely to be self-confident, effective in work and social situations, and comfortable in their relationships. Those who are dissatisfied tend to be self-conscious, inhibited, and less effective in activities.

Plastic surgery—whether cosmetic or reconstructive—encourages and promotes a strong, positive self-image. Even a small change on the outside can create an extraordinary change on the inside, allowing an individual's self-confidence to flourish.

Because the changes resulting from plastic surgery are often dramatic and permanent, it's important that you have a clear understanding of how surgery might make you feel—long before a procedure is scheduled.

This text will provide you with a basic understanding of the psychological issues involved with plastic surgery. It can't answer all your questions, since your individual circumstances and your self-image must be considered. Ask your surgeon if there is anything you don't understand about the possible psychological aspects and effects of your planned procedure.

American Society of Plastic Surgeons, reprinted from The Plastic Surgery Information Service at www.plasticsurgery.org. © 1994; reprinted with permission.

Appropriate Candidates for Surgery

If you are considering plastic surgery, you must be honest with yourself. Exactly why do you want surgery? And, what are your goals for surgery—what do you expect plastic surgery to do for you?

There are two categories of patients who are good candidates for surgery. The first includes patients with a strong self-image, who are bothered by a physical characteristic that they'd like to improve or change. After surgery, these patients feel good about the results and maintain a positive image about themselves.

The second category includes patients who have a physical defect or cosmetic flaw that has diminished their self-esteem over time. These patients may adjust rather slowly after surgery, as rebuilding confidence takes time. However, as they adjust, these patients' self-image is strengthened, sometimes dramatically.

It's important to remember that plastic surgery can create both physical changes and changes in self-esteem. If you are seeking surgery with the hope of influencing a change in someone other than yourself, you might end up disappointed. It's possible that friends and loved ones will respond positively to your change in appearance and self-confidence, however understand and accept that plastic surgery will not cause dramatic changes in people other than you.

Inappropriate Candidates for Surgery

Not everyone is an appropriate candidate for plastic surgery, despite physical indications which are ideal for any given procedure. Experienced plastic surgeons can usually identify troubled patients during a consultation. Sometimes, plastic surgeons will decline to operate on these individuals. Other times, they may recommend psychological counseling to ensure that the patient's desire for an appearance change isn't part of an emotional problem that no amount of surgery can fix. If your plastic surgeon recommends counseling for you, feel free to ask your surgeon how he or she expects the sessions to help you.

Though there are exceptions, individuals who may be advised to seek counseling prior to any consideration of surgery include:

- Patients in crisis, such as those who are going through divorce, the death of a spouse, or the loss of a job. These patients may be seeking to achieve goals that cannot be obtained through an appearance change—goals that relate to overcoming crisis through an unrelated change in appearance is not the solution. Rather, a patient must first work through the crisis.

- Patients with unrealistic expectations, such as those who insist on having a celebrity's nose, with the hope that they may acquire a celebrity lifestyle; patients who want to be restored to their original "perfection" following a severe accident or a serious illness; or patients who wish to find the youth of many decades past.

- Impossible-to-please patients, such as individuals who consult with surgeon after surgeon, seeking the answers they want to hear. These patients hope for a cure to a problem which is not primarily, or not at all physical.

- Patients who are obsessed with a very minor defect, and may believe that once their defect is fixed, life will be perfect. Born perfectionists may be suitable candidates for surgery, as long as they are realistic enough to understand that surgical results may not precisely match their goals.

- Patients who have a mental illness, and exhibit delusional or paranoid behavior, may also be poor candidates for surgery. Surgery may be appropriate in these cases if it is determined that the patient's goals for surgery are not related to the psychosis. In these cases, a plastic surgeon may work closely with the patient's psychiatrist.

The Consultation

During your initial consultation, your plastic surgeon will seek honest answers to how you feel about your appearance, how you believe others see you, and how you'd prefer to look and feel. Honesty, with yourself and with the surgeon is essential. It's important that you set aside any awkwardness you might feel, and speak candidly about the changes you'd like to see. At the end of the consultation, you should feel confident that you and your surgeon understand each other completely.

Also, it is unwise to stress a minor functional problem if your true desire is to have an improved appearance. A patient who pretends to be seeking relief for a functional problem may confuse the surgeon about that patient's true goals for surgery.

Often these patients stress a functional problem with the hope of obtaining insurance coverage for the procedure even though a functional problem does not exist. If your goals for surgery are not clearly communicated to your surgeon, you may not be satisfied with the final result.

Plastic Surgery for Children

Parents may face considerable confusion and anguish in making surgical choices for their children, or when their children show a desire to change or correct a physical characteristic.

For reconstructive procedures such as cleft lip and palate repair, or infant skull surgery, the benefits of early treatment are usually quite clear. Parents typically meet with surgeons, psychologists, and other specialists who provide abundant assurances that surgery is the best choice for their child.

However, in elective procedures like otoplasty (ear pinning), the choices may be more indefinite. If the child doesn't seem to notice that he or she looks "different," parents may be advised not to force the issue of surgery. However, if the child is being teased or feels he or she doesn't belong, parents should probably consider surgery for the emotional health and self-esteem of the child. It's important to follow the recommendation of a pediatrician and to consider the feelings of the child and the parents.

Certain cosmetic surgery procedures may also be of significant psychological benefit for some teenagers, provided that he or she is well-adjusted, both socially and emotionally. Parents need to keep in mind that feelings about self-image tend to change with maturity, and that cosmetic surgery should never be forced on a teenager, nor should a teenager force an issue which a surgeon feels is not an appropriate cause for surgery.

Timing of Surgery

Plastic surgery procedures can impose stress in addition to that which we encounter on a daily basis, both on the body and mind. It's important that surgery is timed at a point when you don't feel exceptional stress, or physical or emotional burden.

To make sure you're emotionally prepared for surgery, your plastic surgeon may ask some rather personal questions about your relationships, home life, work problems, and other private matters. Once again, honesty is essential. In general, surgery should not be scheduled during a time of high activity or emotional upheaval. Patients who go into surgery feeling preoccupied or pressured with other matters may face longer and more difficult recovery periods.

Adjusting to Change

It may take a while before you find you have emotionally recovered from surgery and have adjusted completely to change. This is particularly true if the procedure you've had has significantly changed your body image. If you're planning a relatively straight forward cosmetic procedure like chemical peel or eyelid surgery, you'll probably adjust easily to your new look. Your reflection in the mirror will be a familiar one—a refreshed, younger-looking you.

However, if you plan to have breast surgery, nose surgery, or another procedure that may involve a dramatic body change, the post-operative adjustment period may take longer. Until you learn to accept your redefined body image as your own, your reflection may seem somewhat unfamiliar.

Getting the Support You Need

It's essential to have someone to help you, both physical and emotionally, during your recovery period. Even the most independent patient needs some emotional support after surgery. Remember, during the first week of recovery, you'll have days when you'll feel depressed and look swollen, bruised, and rather unpleasant.

Be sure to select a support person who will be just that—supportive. Graciously decline offers of help from those who may be critical of your decision to have surgery or may be overly troubled by your temporarily bruised and swollen appearance.

Also keep in mind that it's not unusual for a well-meaning friend or relative to say "I liked the way you were before," or "You didn't really need surgery." Comments such as these may cause or worsen feelings of regret or self-doubt, particularly during the early recovery period. Rely on your support person or your surgeon to help you though these difficult times—and try to focus on the reasons you decided to have surgery in the first place.

Coping with Post-Operative Depression

After surgery, most patients experience mild feelings of unhappiness. However, for an unlucky few, post-operative depression may be more severe.

Post-surgery let downs usually set in about three days after surgery—at a point when you may be regaining some of your physical stamina, but your post-operative appearance has not yet begun to improve. In fact, some plastic surgeons call this condition "the Third-Day Blues." It may last anywhere from a few days to several weeks. This emotional let down may be caused by stress, exhaustion, metabolic changes, or the frustration of waiting for results to appear. Depression may be especially stressful for patients undergoing staged procedures, who must cope with an unfinished "interval image" until the final stage of surgery is complete. Patients who are most vulnerable to depression are those who have a history of depression, or who were already somewhat depressed before surgery.

Knowing what to expect in the post-operative period may help you cope better in the days following surgery. It's helpful to remember that the depression usually lifts naturally within about a week. Brisk walks, light social activity, and small outings may help you shake the blues faster.

Handling the Critics

The results of your surgery are likely to elicit some comment from friends and family members—and usually, it's not all positive. If you've had purely cosmetic surgery, you may be criticized for being foolish or frivolous. If your surgery involved changing an ethnic trait, you may be accused of trying to deny your cultural heritage. And, if you changed a family trait, prepare yourself for some surprised or disapproving glances. You may even get the cold shoulder from close friends who feel threatened by your improved appearance.

Some patients find it's helpful to arm themselves with a standard reply to post-operative criticism, such as, "This is something I did for myself—and I'm very happy with my results."

Remember, if you are content with how the results of plastic surgery make you look and feel, then the procedure was indeed a success.

Additional information on plastic surgery is available from the Plastic Surgery Information Service web site at www.plasticsurgery.org or call (800) 635-0635.

Chapter 5

Aesthetic Plastic Surgery for Teenagers

As aesthetic (cosmetic) plastic surgery gains wider acceptance as a method for enhancing body image and self-confidence, it is being considered at an increasingly younger age. For many teens, this option offers significant benefits and little potential for harm. However, for those who lack the necessary emotional and physical maturity, the opposite is true.

Questions to Ask

Parents are often uncertain about the advisability of aesthetic plastic surgery for teenagers under the age of 18. The American Society of Plastic and Reconstructive Surgeons and the American Society for Aesthetic Plastic Surgery offer these guidelines for parents, including these questions they should ask themselves and their teen:

- Who originally suggested that aesthetic surgery be performed? Ideally, the teen should be the one to voice the desire for surgery, and the request should be expressed more than once over a period of time. A suggestion by a parent that cosmetic surgery is needed could create insecurity where none previously existed, leaving the teen feeling unloved or "flawed." If parents suspect that their child is suppressing negative feelings about a body

"Aesthetic Plastic Surgery for Teenagers: When is it Appropriate?" in *Plastic Surgical Nursing*, Summer 1997, vol. 17, no. 2, p. 91(2). ©1997. American Society of Plastic and Reconstructive Surgical Nurses; reprinted with permission.

feature, "leading" questions can be asked, such as, "If you could change one thing about yourself, what would it be?"

• What does the youth expect surgery will do for him or her? If a young person asks for surgery, or complains about an unattractive body feature, find out exactly what it is that he or she doesn't like, what effect it has had, how he or she thinks a change would improve the body feature, and how long he or she has been feeling this way. Parents should watch for signs that their child is blaming a less-than-perfect nose or chin for a lack of popularity, a soured love relationship, or similar problem. If such an individual were to have aesthetic surgery, only to find that he or she still was not popular, the effects on the youth's self-esteem could be far more serious than the original problem.

• Has the teen been consistent in his or her likes and dislikes? Teens who change their fashion preferences quite frequently— such as those who constantly experiment with new glasses or hair color—are often poor candidates for aesthetic surgery. Chances are high that they will not remain satisfied with the results of surgery either—but, unlike hair color, the change is permanent.

When talking with their child, parents should keep in mind that early in childhood, the desire to be just like everyone else is very strong. However, as children enter late adolescence, individuality is more valued and is accepted more comfortably. Simple words that reassure the teen of a parent's love, and that help him or her realize that everyone has similar experiences during childhood, are sometimes enough consolation.

On the other hand, parents should be careful not to discount their child's feelings, particularly when they are expressed repeatedly in realistic terms. This is especially true when children complain about a large nose or other body feature inherited from a parent, who often has learned to be comfortable with the characteristic or views it as mark of family "identity." Waiting too long before "giving in" could cause the child years of unnecessary emotional trauma.

Seek Advice

When parents are in doubt about a child's need for aesthetic surgery, the advice of a pediatrician or plastic surgeon can help put the issue into perspective. When selecting a plastic surgeon, parents and their children may want to interview several physicians who are certified by the American Board of Plastic Surgery to find one with whom they feel a strong rapport. Any physician who lacks formal training in plastic surgery, who tries to "sell" a parent or teen on a particular procedure, or who fails to discuss possible complications should be avoided.

Names of certified plastic surgeons who perform the desired procedure in a specific locale can be obtained by calling the toll-free telephone number of the Cosmetic Plastic Surgery Referral Line, 1-888-ASAPS-11 (1-888-272-7711).

The plastic surgeon should evaluate the prospective patient's perception of his or her problem, as well as the desired results. During this interview, it is often advisable for the plastic surgeon to talk with the prospective patient separately from the parents. This removes the influence of any potential parental pressure and allows the teen or adolescent to speak more freely about potentially embarrassing issues. Because teens often have fragile body images and may not cope well with complications after surgery, these possibilities should also be thoroughly discussed during the consultation.

Finally, an assessment of the prospective patient's physical maturity is essential, since operating on a feature that has not yet fully developed could interfere with growth or negate the benefits of surgery in later years. The following recommendations are offered for patients under the age of 18:

Usually Inappropriate

- *Breast enlargement*. This procedure is rarely recommended before the age of 18, due to the likelihood of late development that could result in a significantly larger size than desired.

- *Liposuction*. Teens often seek liposuction as a "cure" for unwanted baby fat, particularly in the face. Although the procedure will usually provide the sought-after look, the effects are frequently temporary. Later in life, as aging occurs, the absence of fat may result in sagging skin and sunken-in cheeks, causing individuals to look older than they actually are. By waiting a few years, teens often find that the "baby fat" that gives their faces a round look disappears on its own.

- *Cheek implants*. The results are usually very subtle and the desired benefits must be evaluated carefully.

Usually Appropriate

- *Rhinoplasty (nose reshaping)*. This is the most common aesthetic procedure requested by teens. It can be performed when the nose has completed 90 percent of its growth, which can occur as young as 13 or 14 in girls and 15 or 16 in boys.

- *Otoplasty (in which protruding ears are "pinned" back)*. This can be performed in children as young as five years old.

- *Breast reduction*. This procedure can help girls as young as 16 who are embarrassed by overly large breasts, and who may be experiencing symptoms such as shoulder pains and breathing difficulty.

- *Correction of breast asymmetry*. When one breast significantly differs from the other in terms of either size or shape, surgery can help girls as young as 16 years.

- *Treatment for gynecomastia*. Excessive breast development on one or both sides is often experienced by teenage boys. In some, the condition is slight and disappears on its own after a short while; however, for others it persists and can become a significant psychosocial problem. Excess tissue can be removed in boys as young as 16.

- *Chin augmentation*. This procedure can be appropriate when a teen has reached the age of 15. A chin implant is often needed to correct problems blamed on the nose, and is frequently inserted in conjunction with a rhinoplasty.

Most experts agree that, for carefully selected teenage patients, aesthetic plastic surgery can have a positive impact on physical and emotional development. Parents and teens must be willing to talk openly about their feelings and expectations regarding aesthetic surgery. The appropriateness of any aesthetic surgery procedure is a highly individual matter that should be determined with the guidance of a board-certified plastic surgeon.

Both the American Society of Plastic and Reconstructive Surgeons and the American Society for Aesthetic Plastic Surgery require active members to be certified by the American Board of Plastic Surgery. Consumers wishing to receive a copy of this statement, as well as the names of certified plastic surgeons in their area, may call 1-888-ASAPS-11 (1-888-272-7711).

Note: This document was originally released by The American Society of Plastic and Reconstructive Surgeons and the American Society for Aesthetic Plastic Surgery in September 1990; it has been revised to include information available as of December 1994.

Chapter 6

Realistic Motivations, Expectations Crucial to Surgical Success

Why do you want to have this surgery? What do you hope the procedure will do for you?

Don't be surprised when your facial plastic surgeon asks these questions. It's a standard part of the initial consultation, because facial plastic surgeons know how important it is for patients to have appropriate motivations for seeking surgery and realistic expectations about what the procedure will accomplish.

Look Good, Feel Good

Facial plastic surgery is one of the tools available to help people look their best. Health professionals today recognize the link between physical appearance and self-esteem. Psychologists point out that a desire for an attractive appearance is a sign of good mental health, because attention to one's looks demonstrates healthy self-esteem.

People who look good tend to feel better about themselves. People treat them with greater respect, and that starts an upward spiral of success. An attractive appearance is no guarantee of happiness, however. And while a pleasing appearance is one factor in developing healthy self-esteem, it is not the only one.

Facial plastic surgeons agree that the best candidates for a surgical procedure are individuals who already have a strong self-concept.

American Academy of Facial Plastic and Reconstructive Surgery, *Today* newsletter, First Quarter 1998, Vol. 12, No. 1. © 1998, American Academy of Facial and Reconstructive Plastic Surgeons; reprinted with permission.

They like themselves, and know exactly what they want to accomplish. They are seeking facial plastic surgery to improve their appearance, but they are not expecting it to change their lives.

Your Consultation Visit

When you first meet with the surgeon, you should be prepared to explain exactly what you think is wrong with your face and what you would like the surgery to accomplish. The problem may seem obvious to you, but the surgeon will want you to describe it in your own words and tell why you want to make a change.

The surgeon will probe into your attitudes because realistic expectations are important if you are to obtain a successful result. Facial plastic surgery can improve appearance, but it does not yield perfection. Patients whose expectations are unrealistic or unattainable may have difficulty adjusting to their new appearance, or they may be unable to accept the natural effects of surgery. Any facial plastic surgery procedure inevitably involves some discomfort and a period of swelling or discoloration. Patients must understand the risks and be strongly motivated to follow through with appropriate postoperative care.

Motivations for Surgery

So why are you having surgery? If you are like most facial plastic surgery patients, your primary motivation is a desire to look younger. Dissatisfaction with a facial feature and a desire to improve one's outer appearance are the next most commonly cited reasons, according to a survey conducted by the American Academy of Facial Plastic and Reconstructive Surgery.

Facial plastic surgery is on the upswing, with well over a million aesthetic procedures performed each year. People from every walk of life are opting for nose surgery, facelifts, browlifts, eyelid surgery, hair replacement procedures, and other techniques for improving their appearance. They are finding that facial plastic surgery offers an affordable and realistic option for correcting facial problems.

Surgery Won't Change Your Life

What do you hope surgery will accomplish? If you say that you hope it will help you look your best, you are right on target for a successful experience. It's a mistake to think facial plastic surgery will fix what's wrong in your life. It won't help you salvage a failed relationship or get a promotion at work. Not surprisingly, surgeons hesitate to operate on people whose reasons for wanting surgery are inappropriate and who are seeking more than surgery can do.

Still Myself, Only Better

Facial plastic surgery won't put someone else's features on your face. Nor will it make you look just the way you did 20 years ago. What it can do is to improve and harmonize your unique features—and make you look the best you can be.

As one satisfied facial plastic surgery patient commented, My friends say I look great, but no one has any idea that I had surgery! It didn't change the way I look—I'm still myself, only better.

Chapter 7

Complications of
Laser Resurfacing

The Utra Pulse carbon dioxide laser has rapidly become an important tool for the rejuvenation of facial skin. Wrinkles, precancerous lesions, hyperpigmentation, dermatochalasis, acne scarring, as well as sun-damaged skin can be effectively treated using the new group of CO_2 lasers. These lasers are truly remarkable technological advancements in the field of anti-aging surgery. The laser affords significant benefits over traditional resurfacing and incisional techniques such as dermabrasion, chemical peel, and blepharoplasty, especially in the areas of control, safety, customization, and hemostasis. The advantages of laser technology are clearly noted by practitioners and patients. It is important to prevent potential complications from the laser and recognize potential complications that can lead to scarring. This article reviews complications known to date. See Tables 7.1. and 7.2. for a summary.

"Complications of Laser Resurfacing," by Brooke R. Seckel; Laurie Watson, in *Plastic Surgical Nursing*, Fall 1997 vol. 17, no. 3, p. 138(7). ©1997 American Society of Plastic and Reconstructive Surgical Nurses; reprinted with permission.

Table 7.1. Complications of Laser Resurfacing—Recognition, Management, and Prevention

Complication	Prevention	Symptoms
1. Eye Injury	Scleral Shields	Eye pain, Changes in corneal surface
2. Hypertrophic Scar	Do not go too deep, Avoid Infection, Avoid maceration, Pre-Operative skin care	Early Palpable Induration
3. Ectropion	Check for Eyelid laxity Canthoplasty (Jelks via upper lid incision), Conservative Resurfacing	Lax Lid, Scleral Show
4. Prolonged Redness	Pre-treat Skin, Do not go too deep	Skin erythema
5. Milia	Pre-treat Skin, Avoid heavy ointments	White pustules
6. Hyperpigmentation	Patient Selection (Less than type IV), Pre-treat skin	Skin color change
7. Hypopigmentation	Patient Selection (Less than type IV), Do not go too deep	Skin color loss
8. Herpes Simplex	History, Prophylactic, Valtrex 500 mg 2 p.o., t.i.d. 1 day pre-op and 7-10 days post-op	Pain, Redness, Full Thickness, Tzanck Smear
9. Bacterial or Fungal Infection	Prophylactic Antibiotic, Eryc 500mg b.i.d., High index suspicion, Avoid maceration, Avoid eschar, Treat like burn wound	Pain, Fever, Exudate, Thick eschar, Kohs prep (Fungus), Gram stain, Tzanck smear (Herpes)

Table 7.2. Management of Complications.

Complication	Management
1. Eye Injury	Consult Ophthalmologist
2. Hypertrophic Scar	Aggressive treatment (10 day), Temovate
3. Ectropion	Canthopexy-Pre-op, Massage, Flexzan, Steroids (topical or injection), Lubricate eye
4. Prolonged Redness	Hydrocortisone cream
5. Milia	Open with extractor, Hydrocortisone cream, Hema Tech Smoothing Gel
6. Hyperpigmentation	Bleaching cream All recover
7. Hypopigmentation	None
8. Herpes Simplex	Valtrex 500 mg 2 p.o. t.i.d. 1 day pre-op and 7-10 days post-op,
9. Bacterial or Fungal Infection	Removal all dressings, Culture for fungi and bacteria, Keep wound clean, Vinegar H_2O wet to dry, Diflucan (anti-fungal) 150 mg 2 p.o. day 1, then p.o. every day, Duricef 500mg p.o. q.i.d. Keflex 500 mg, p.o. q.i.d.

Chapter 8

Surgical Risks of Breast Implants

In addition to the risks of anesthesia and surgery in general, there are complications that may result from any surgical procedure that places a foreign object (including a breast implant) in the body. It is not known how frequently the following occur, but the frequency is dependent on both patient and surgical factors.

- **Hematoma** is a collection of blood or a blood clot from a leak in a blood vessel that may form within hours after surgery in the pocket where the implant has been placed. If this happens, swelling, pain and bruising may result. Large hematomas may have to be drained surgically for proper healing. Surgical drainage may cause scarring, which is minimal in most women.

- **Infection** is a risk associated with any surgical procedure, including insertion or removal of a breast implant, and requires immediate medical attention. Infections occur in a few percent of women receiving implants. Most infections occur soon after surgery, but they can happen, although rarely, much later. If you notice signs of infection such as pain, redness, swelling, tenderness, fever, or drainage at the operative site, call your surgeon immediately. Infection after any type of surgery can be serious. If the infection does not subside promptly with the appropriate treatment, removal of the implant may be necessary.

U.S. Food and Drug Administration, Office of Consumer Affairs, reprinted from www.fda.gov/oca/breastimplants/birisk.html, revised/posted 12/8/98.

If that happens, a new device can usually be implanted after the infection has completely cleared.

A few cases of toxic shock syndrome related to breast implants (and not related to menstruation or tampon use) have been reported.[1]

Other Implant-Related Risks

In addition to the surgical risks discussed above, other risks are associated specifically with breast implants. The surgeon should discuss these with you well in advance of surgery.

If possible, a month before the surgery, ask your surgeon for full information on the risks associated with breast implants, including:

- the patient package insert for your specific type of implant(s),

- the patient information sheet for women considering saline-filled implants, and

- a copy of the informed consent form usually given to the patient prior to surgery for either saline or silicone gel-filled implants.

The adverse effects from breast implants fall into two categories. The first consists of **known risks** that are clearly associated with these devices. The second consists of **problems that have not been scientifically shown to be associated with breast implants but have been reported** by some women who have them. Scientists are conducting research to determine if an association does exist between these reported problems and breast implants.

Known Implant-Related Risks

Additional Surgery

Additional surgery is a risk for women with either silicone gel-filled or saline-filled implants. Surgery may be needed to treat a serious problem with the implant, or to remove a ruptured implant and, if desired, replace it. A recent study found that 24 percent of women with breast implants experience adverse events resulting in surgery during the first five years after implantation (silicone and saline implants were combined). The likelihood of needing additional surgery was greater for reconstruction than for augmentation. According to this study, women getting breast implants for reconstruction can expect about a one-in-three chance of needing a second surgery within five years; women getting breast implants for augmentation can expect about a one-in-eight chance of needing a second surgery within five years. Additional surgeries may result in (additional) loss of breast tissue.[2]

Rupture, Deflation, and Leakage

Breast implants **are not lifetime devices** and cannot be expected to last forever. Some implants deflate (or rupture) in the first few months after being implanted and some deflate after several years; yet others are intact 10 or more years after the surgery.

- Magnetic resonance imaging (MRI) may be used for evaluating patients with suspected rupture, deflation or leakage. Discuss this and other options with your doctor.

- In addition to the length of time the implant has been in the body, the chance of rupture also increases with injury to the breast. Closed capsulotomy, a technique used to break capsular contracture by squeezing the breast, has also been implicated as a possible cause of breast implant rupture; closed capsulotomy is not recommended by breast implant manufacturers.

Saline-Filled Implants

Saline-filled implants may be more vulnerable to damage and deflation than gel-filled implants. When a saline-filled implant deflates, it usually happens quickly. Surgery is then required to remove the ruptured implant and replace it, if desired. Since salt water is naturally present in the body, the body will absorb the leaked saline solution from the implant instead of reacting to it as foreign matter.

- The rupture rate for saline implants varies and seems to be dependent on many factors, including manufacturing quality standards and length of time since manufacture.

- It is not known when deflation is most likely to happen. The implant may break due to injury to the breast or normal aging of the implant, releasing the salt water filling.

Silicone Gel-Filled Implants

When silicone gel-filled implants rupture, some women may notice decreased breast size, nodules, uneven appearance of the breasts, pain or tenderness, tingling, swelling, numbness, burning, or changes in sensation. Other women may experience a rupture and not notice any differences. Plastic surgeons usually recommend explantation if the implant has ruptured, even if the silicone is still enclosed within the scar tissue capsule, because the device is no longer working as intended. If you are considering the removal of an implant and the implantation of another one, be sure to discuss the benefits and risks with your doctor.

- The rate at which silicone gel-filled implants rupture is uncertain. However, using different methods for detection, published studies suggest between 5 and 51 percent of women experience rupture, an enormous range. A study of screening mammograms suggested that 5 percent of **asymptomatic** women had experienced "silent rupture" of their implants. Mammography is of **limited value in detecting implant rupture**. The mammogram readings of rupture were not confirmed by surgical removal of the implant. Robinson et al. studied 300 women who had their implants for one to 25 years and had their implants removed for a variety of reasons.[4] They found visible signs of ruptures in 51 percent of the women studied. Severe silicone leakage—silicone outside the implant without visible tears or holes—was seen in another 20 percent. Robinson et al. also noted that the probability of rupture increases as the implant ages and recommended removal of all gel-filled implants preferably before eight years of implantation.

- A silicone gel-filled implant may rupture but stay contained within the fibrous capsule the body has made around the implant. Silicone gel which escapes the fibrotic capsule surrounding the implant may migrate away from the breast. The free silicone may cause lumps called granulomas to form in the breast or other tissues where the silicone has migrated, such as the chest wall, armpit, arm or abdomen. Some studies indicate that silicone may escape the capsule in 10-20 percent of rupture cases.[5]

Other Known Risks (For all Breast Implants)

- **Capsular contracture** is a tightening of scar tissue around the implant. This can sometimes cause pain, hardening of the breast, or changes in breast appearance. Although it seems to occur to some extent in most women with breast implants, there are no reliable data on how often this happens.[6] If these changes are severe, more surgery may be needed to correct or remove the implants.

- **Calcium deposits** may form in surrounding tissue, and may cause pain and hardening of the scar tissue. In some cases, these deposits may need to be surgically removed.

- **Changes in nipple or breast sensation** may result from the surgery. These changes may be temporary or permanent. They may affect sexual response and the response of the nipple during breast feeding. A woman whose nipple is removed as part of her mastectomy will not have the ability to nurse.

- **Interference with mammogram readings** can occur with breast implants. This interference may delay or hinder the early detection of breast cancer by hiding suspicious lesions. Implants increase the technical difficulty of taking and reading mammograms. It is important that a woman with breast tissue and a breast implant undergo mammography to detect breast cancer.

- **Mammography requires severe breast compression that could contribute to implant rupture.** Special techniques are used **to reduce the risk of implant rupture during this compression, and to maximize visualization of the breast tissue during mammography. These techniques are called breast** implant displacement views, Eklund displacement views, or Eklund views, after the physician who developed them. Women with implants should always inform the **receptionist or scheduler** that they have breast implants when making an appointment for mammography and **tell** the radiologic technologist about the presence of implants **before** mammography is performed. This is to make sure that the technologists use these special displacement techniques and take extra care when compressing the breasts to avoid rupturing the implant.

The displacement procedure involves pushing the implant back and gently pulling the breast tissue into view. Several factors affect the success of this special technique in imaging the breast tissue in women with breast implants. Therefore, the location of the implant, the degree (hardness) of the capsular contracture, the size of the breast tissue compared to the implant and other factors may affect how well the breast tissue can be imaged.

Also, a radiologist may find it difficult to distinguish calcium deposits in the scar tissue around the implant from a breast tumor when he or she is interpreting the mammogram. Occasionally, it is necessary to remove and examine a small amount of tissue (biopsy) to see whether or not it is cancerous. This can frequently be done without removing the implant.

- **Shifting of the implant:** Sometimes an implant may shift from its original position, giving the breasts an unnatural look and possibly causing pain and discomfort. An implant may become visible at the surface of the breast as a result of the device pushing through the layers of skin. Further surgery is needed to correct this problem. Placing the implant beneath the muscle may help to minimize this problem.

- **Granulomas:** These are non-cancerous lumps that can form when your normal body cells surround the foreign material such as silicone and form lumps. These need to be evaluated by your physician to tell them apart from lumps that might be cancerous and may require a biopsy.

- **Other problems with appearance** could include incorrect implant size, visible scars, uneven appearance, and wrinkling of the implant. An implant might break through the skin, particularly if you have very thin breast tissue over the implant. If your implant has a valve, you also might be able to feel the valve of the implant with your hand. **Repeated surgeries** to improve the appearance of the breasts and/or to remove (**explant**) ruptured or deflated prostheses may result in a **dissatisfactory cosmetic outcome**. Women should consider these issues when deciding to have breast implants and carefully discuss their expected cosmetic results with their surgeon prior to surgery.

- **Other potential complications** include breast pain and delayed wound healing.

- **Non-medical considerations** include costs which may or may not be covered by your insurance, your confidentiality for participation in a clinical trial, and the legal disposition of your implant(s) from the manufacturer as a result of a need for removal and your participation in the clinical trial.

Notes

[1]Poblete JV, Rodgers JA, Wolfort, FG. Toxic shock syndrome as a complication of breast prostheses. *Plast Reconstr Surg*. Dec 96(7): 1702-8.

[2]Gabriel SE et al. Complications leading to surgery after breast implantation. NEJM 1997: 336:679-682.

[4]Robinson OG, Bradley EL, Wilson DS. Analysis of explanted silicone implants: A report of 300 patients. *Ann Plast Surg* 1995: 34:1-7.

[5]Vinnik CA. Migratory silicon—clinical aspects. *Silicone in Medical Devices—Conference Proceedings*. 1991 February 1-2; Baltimore, MD: U.S. Department of Health and Human Services, FDA Publication No. 92-4249 (p 59-67).

[6]Burkhardt BR. Capsular contracture: Hard breasts, soft data. *Clinics in Plastic Surgery* 1988: 15:521-532.

Part Three

Plastic Surgery
Techniques and Tools

Chapter 9

What Is Laser?

Laser stands for Light Amplification by the Stimulated Emission of Radiation. Lasers work by producing an intense beam of bright light that travels in one direction. This laser beam can cut, seal or vaporize skin tissue and blood vessels. The laser has the unique ability to produce one specific color (wavelength) of light which can be varied in its intensity and pulse duration. Ordinary light from non-laser sources is composed of many different colors and appears white. The wavelength and power output of a particular laser determines its medical application.

When the laser light is directed at skin tissue, its light energy is absorbed by water or pigments found in the skin. Water is found in large amounts in all living cells. Pigments of the skin include hemoglobin, a protein that makes blood red, and melanin, the tan or brown colored pigment. All three absorb laser light of different colors.

What Are the Benefits of Laser Surgery?

Lasers may offer you and your dermatologic surgeon the following general benefits:

- Improved therapeutic results,
- Reduced risk of infection,

American Society for Dermatologic Surgery, Form No. #002 1996, Rev. 12/ 1997. © 1995-1999; reprinted with permission.

- Relatively "bloodless" surgery,
- Precisely controlled surgery which limits injury to normal skin,
- An alternative to traditional, scalpel surgery, in some cases,
- Potentially less scarring, in some cases, and
- Safe and effective out-patient, same-day surgery for many skin conditions.

What Type of Laser Should Be Used?

In dermatology, many different types of lasers are presently being used to treat a variety of skin conditions, growths and cosmetic complaints. Further, no single laser is currently capable of treating all skin conditions, and some lasers have only limited usefulness in dermatologic applications. In addition, certain lasers can be tuned to a variety of colors of light or coupled to a robotized scanning device to expand their clinical effectiveness.

Your dermatologic surgeon will carefully evaluate your particular problem and then suggest the appropriate type of laser system that might be useful for therapy.

Who Is Qualified to Perform Laser Surgery?

Experts in skin care, dermatologic surgeons have extensive experience with laser surgery and were among the first specialists to use lasers for treating a variety of skin disorders. In fact, many of the latest advances in laser technology were pioneered and refined by dermatologic surgeons. Since results are often technique-sensitive, it's important to select a dermatologic surgeon with laser expertise.

Common Lasers Used in Dermatology

The Carbon Dioxide (CO_2) Laser

The CO_2 laser emits a colorless infrared light which is highly absorbed by water-containing tissue like the skin. This laser system can be used in several ways: "focused" for cutting skin without bleeding; "defocused" for superficially vaporizing skin; and "super pulsed" for facial resurfacing.

By delivering very powerful, rapid pulsing or scanning of the CO_2 laser beam, dermatologic surgeons are able to peel and resurface the facial skin for cosmetic improvement while minimizing damage or scarring surrounding skin. Sometimes referred to as "laserbrasion," this technique removes fine lines and wrinkles of the face, smoothes acne scars and rejuvenates aging and sun-damaged skin as it gently smoothes and precisely contours the skin surface.

If the CO_2 laser's energy is defocused and not continuous (pulsed), a larger spot of light is created which is less intense. With this modification, the dermatologic surgeon can remove or vaporize thin layers from the skin surface without penetrating the deeper layers. This technique is particularly useful in treating warts, shallow tumors and certain precancerous conditions.

When the CO_2 laser energy is continuous and focused into a small spot of light, the beam is able to cut the skin. As an alternative to traditional scalpel surgery, the laser helps to limit blood flow during the treatment and reduce post-operative swelling. The carbon dioxide laser is used in this way to remove skin cancers, to treat a variety of nonvascular and pigmented lesions and for eyelid operations. This technique is also used to remove warts and for some surgical incisions.

The Erbium (Er):YAG Laser

The erbium:YAG laser produces laser energy in a wavelength that gently penetrates the skin, is readily absorbed by water (a major component of tissue cells), and scatters the heat effects of the laser light. These unique properties allow dermatologic surgeons to remove thin layers of skin tissue with exquisite precision while minimizing damage to surrounding skin.

The Er:YAG is commonly used for skin resurfacing in patients who have superficial to moderate facial wrinkles, mild surface scars or splotchy skin discolorations. Skin rejuvenation with the Er:YAG laser offers the benefits of reduced redness, decreased side effects and rapid healing compared to some other lasers.

The Argon Laser

The argon laser emits a blue-green colored light which is absorbed by hemoglobin in blood cells. When hemoglobin absorbs the laser energy, it is converted to heat. The heat damages and seals the blood vessels, causing them to disintegrate and be reabsorbed into the body.

Because of this selective absorption of laser light by hemoglobin, the argon laser is most often used to treat blood vessel disorders and growths, especially those that are raised and bluish-red in color. The argon laser can flatten and lighten these types of growths with little risk of scarring. Specifically, it is capable of treating port wine stains, red birthmarks, hemangiomas (malformations of blood veins in the skin), enlarged blood vessels and the red-nose syndrome that results from acne rosacea or nasal surgery.

Table 9.1. Skin Conditions and Lasers Used

SKIN CONDITION	LASER SYSTEM
Wrinkles and lines	Carbon Dioxide Erbium:YAG
Superficial Brown Pigmented Lesions	Q-switched Alexandrite Argon Carbon Dioxide Copper Vapor Krypton KTP Q-switched Nd:YAG Q-switched Ruby
Deep Pigmented Lesions	Q-switched Ruby Q-switched Nd:YAG Q-switched Alexandrite
Scars and stretch marks	Carbon Dioxide Pulsed Dye
Tattoos	Q-switched Alexandrite Carbon Dioxide Q-switched Nd:YAG Q-switched Ruby
Vascular Lesions	Argon Argon-pumped Tunable Dye Copper Vapor Pulsed Dye Krypton KTP
Warts	Carbon Dioxide Pulsed Dye
Hair Removal	Long-pulsed Ruby Q-switched Nd:YAG Long-pulsed Alexandrite Intense Pulsed Light Sources

The Yellow Light Lasers

Through the use of an organic dye, short pulses of yellow colored light are produced. A popular yellow light laser is the pulsed dye laser, which uses a camera-like flash to stimulate the dye solution to produce yellow light. Because yellow light is more precisely absorbed by the hemoglobin than other colors, these lasers are effective in the treatment of blood vessel disorders, such as port wine stains, red birthmarks, enlarged blood vessels, rosacea, hemangiomas and red-nose syndrome. Like the other lasers, yellow light lasers can be used with minimal risk of scarring from treatment, making them safe and effective in the treatment of infants and children.

Some yellow light laser systems can be adjusted to produce multiple colors of light. For instance, the argon-pumped tunable dye laser, though more commonly used to make yellow light, can also be tuned to produce red light. This wavelength is used in an experimental technique known as "photodynamic therapy" for the treatment of skin cancer.

Similarly, the copper vapor laser heats elemental copper to produce both yellow and green colors of light. The uses of the yellow light are similar to those already described. The green light, in contrast, is used for the treatment of benign brown-pigmented lesions, such as cafe-au-lait spots, the "old age" spots commonly found on the backs of the hands, and lentigines or freckles.

Another dual light system is the krypton laser. As a source of yellow light, it treats vascular lesions. When adjusted to produce a green light, the krypton laser can treat brown-pigmented lesions.

The Red Light Lasers

The red light spectrum produced by the ruby laser is emitted in extremely short, high-energy pulses. This type of pulse is possible due to a technique known as Q-switching. The Q-switched ruby laser system was initially used to remove tattoos, particularly amateur tattoos, since it can effectively fade or eliminate the colored pigments with little risk of scarring or damage to the surrounding skin. In addition, this laser is now commonly used to treat many brown-pigmented lesions, such as actinic lentigines, freckles, cafe-au-lait spots and nevus of Ota.

Another laser in the red category is the Q-switched alexandrite laser. Like the ruby laser, its energy is selectively absorbed by melanin, making it effective for tattoo removal and benign brown-pigmented lesions.

Other Lasers

The Q-switched neodymium:YAG (Nd:YAG) laser delivers two different wavelengths of light. One is an invisible infrared light used to remove blue-black tattoos, traumatic tattoos and deep dermal-pigmented lesions, such as nevus of Ota. This laser can also be tuned to produce a green light for the treatment of superficial pigmented lesions like brown spots, as well as orange-red tattoos. In both cases, the Q-switching device emits rapid bursts of the laser beam to the treatment site.

Another laser is the KTP which emits a green light and is capable of treating certain vascular and brown pigmented lesions.

Other Applications: Hair Removal

Laser technology is presently being utilized for efficient and long-lasting body hair removal. Although experts remain uncertain precisely how the treatment works, it appears that the laser energy causes thermal injury to the hair follicle. Several intense pulsed light devices and laser hair-removal systems, such as the long-pulsed ruby laser, the Q-switched Nd:YAG laser, and the long-pulsed alexandrite laser, are being explored by dermatologic surgeons with promising results. In preliminary clinical trials, test sites remained hair-free for up to three months in some cases. While the application of lasers for facial and body hair removal is still in its infancy, dermatologic surgeons are enthusiastic about this treatment and its future.

For More Information

For more information on laser treatments and to obtain a referral list of laser experts in your geographic area, call the American Society for Dermatologic Surgery's toll-free consumer hotline, 1-800-441-2737, during weekday business hours (CST).

The American Society for Dermatologic Surgery (ASDS)

The ASDS provides grants, training and continuing education for its members in new dermatologic surgical techniques and procedures. Represented in the American Medical Association House of Delegates, the Society was formed in 1970 to promote excellence in the subspecialty of dermatologic surgery and to foster the highest standards of patient care. American Society for Dermatologic Surgery, 930 North Meacham Road, Schaumburg, Illinois 60173-6016; Phone: (847) 330-9830 or visit our website at http://www.asds-net.org.

Chapter 10

Combining High-Tech Surgical Techniques for Effective Restorative Facial Surgery

Three-dimensional imaging, Doppler monitoring, microsurgical techniques, and camouflage makeup can be combined to reconstruct faces that have been severely disfigured by burns, trauma, or congenital birth defects. Multi-stage reconstruction uses microvascular free-tissue transfer to replace entire aesthetic units of the face, such as the cheek, neck, nose, lips, or ears. For more than a decade, microvascular flap techniques have been used successfully in breast surgery, neurosurgery, and other surgical subspecialties, but the technique has been underutilized in facial reconstruction.

"Most of my extensively burned patients are in their teens or twenties with five to six decades of productivity ahead of them," indicates plastic surgeon Elliott H. Rose, affiliated with the Mount Sinai Medical Center, New York City. "This newly refined surgical procedure, known as aesthetic facial restoration, allows them to regain a normal appearance, reintegrate into society, and have fulfilling lives."

More commonly, skin grafts have been used to reconstruct facial disfigurement. However, grafts often produce skin that is hard and rigid with a corrugated, thick surface texture. The procedure frequently masks facial animation, leaving an expressionless look.

In a study conducted over a period of eight years, multi-stage reconstruction was performed on 18 burn patients with severely

"Restoring Severely Disfigured Faces: Combining High-Tech Surgical Techniques for Effective Restorative Facial Surgery" in *USA Today (Magazine),* October 1996, vol. 125, no. 2617, p. 8(1). ©1996 Society for the Advancement of Education; reprinted with permission.

disfigured faces. Among the facial areas reconstructed were neck, chin and lower lip, jaw, cheek, nose, upper lip, ear, forehead, and scalp, as well as the periorbital area around the eyes.

Before surgery, high-resolution video imaging was used to plan the procedure and project the desired surgical outcome. Specialized software was used to diagnose and re-create any bone or soft tissue abnormalities and assess the symmetry of the face. A three-dimensional video image of facial architecture was created, and a computer-generated acrylic model of the missing bone was fashioned from the digital data. Then, the actual bone graft was carved to fit the space like the missing piece of a puzzle.

Flaps taken from the forearm, back, or other areas with similar tissue consistency were "pre-patterned" so that they exactly fit the appropriate facial unit with seams falling in the natural creases of the face. Using microsurgical techniques, tiny blood vessels no more than two millimeters in diameter were attached to the facial artery to restore immediate circulation to the flap. Flaps then were "sculpted" to achieve the normal planes and contours of the face. Using the sound waves of a Doppler monitor to locate deep blood vessels, excess tissue was removed from the underside of the newly placed flap to look, feel, and behave like normal facial skin.

After surgical restoration was complete, a makeup specialist evaluated the patients and developed a makeup routine to camouflage the scars and blend the color of the transplanted skin with the rest of the face. A green underbase neutralized the reddish scars, and a hypoallergenic flesh-colored foundation make skin color more even.

"We have only one objective in aesthetically restoring balance and symmetry to the face of these severely burned patients," Rose points out, "and that is to reintegrate them as functioning, productive members of society. The alternative may well be a societal 'drop-out,' recluse, or drug addict."

Chapter 11

New Simulation Software Called Immersive Workbench

The surgeon studies the face of a teenage boy whose upper jaw and cheek were destroyed by cancer years ago. Lifting his gloved right hand, he points to an area just below one of the patient's eyes. As if by magic, an incision appears in the boy's cheek, revealing the area of tissue and bone to be rebuilt. Pointing again, the surgeon begins a complicated procedure for transplanting bone and tissue from the boy's hip to his face.

In the past, plastic surgeons had to be in the operating room to try procedures like these. Now some are using an experimental computer visualization tool called the Immersive Workbench, developed by researchers from Stanford University and National Aeronautics and Space Administration (NASA) Ames Research Center, to plan and practice difficult operations. The software program combines data from computerized axial tomography (CT) scans, magnetic resonance images, and ultrasound to create high-resolution pictures of individual patients and display them in a virtual environment. Unlike other software tools developed to visualize the results of plastic surgery, which rely on standard physical models of men and women, the Immersive Workbench generates images that depict the specific deformities or injuries of particular patients. The latest prototype of the software goes further, letting doctors wearing tracked-shutter glasses

"Practice Makes Perfect (New Surgical Simulation Software Called Immersive Workbench)," by Mark Hodges, in *MIT's Technology Review*, March-April 1998 v101 n2 p17(2). ©1998 Massachusetts Institute of Technology Alumni Association; reprinted with permission.

and special gloves test specific surgical approaches in rapid succession to see which produces the best results.

"The whole idea is to be able to interact with the virtual environment in the same way as you interact with a patient in real life—in a way that requires almost no training for the user," says project director Dr. Michael Stephanides of Stanford University's Division of Plastic Surgery.

The project started in 1991, when Stanford researchers began developing two-dimensional graphic renderings of patients from imaging data. Three years ago, Stephanides asked NASA Ames to create sophisticated software for building three-dimensional patient portraits from data collected in CT scans. At that time, NASA Ames engineers were spending most of their time creating visualizations of biological systems for space-related applications, but the lab's collaboration with Stanford has led to the creation of NASA Ames's Biocomputation Center, a new national center for research in virtual environments for surgical planning.

Plastic surgery offers a particularly rigorous challenge for software engineers and medical researchers developing virtual reality (VR) tools, since computerized renderings of patients must look almost exactly as they do in the real world. It is no small task to display human body parts at the necessary high resolution, says Kevin Montgomery, the leader of the NASA Ames group participating in this project. According to Montgomery, a 3-D rendering of a human face and head contains 8 million tiny image slices that must be updated at a speed of 10 frames per second—processing demands that approach the theoretical limit of current computers; as a result, the NASA Ames researchers had to find ingenious ways to discard much of the raw data from patient images. Nonetheless, Montgomery's group has been able to generate highly resolved images detailing such subtle features as small ridges of tissue, the impression of a vein beneath the skin on a human scalp, and the fine detail of a patient's inner ear.

Doctors have already used the Immersive Workbench to plan some 15 surgeries involving reconstruction of bony defects in the skeleton of the face and skull. But Montgomery and Stephanides caution that the tool is still in the experimental stage. They expect clinical deployment in three to five years, when the next generation of processors and graphics cards makes $10,000 desktop computers as fast and powerful as the $100,000 graphical workstations now needed to run the software. Between now and then, the researchers hope to improve the program by creating a more intuitive graphical user interface, depicting virtual surgical instruments more accurately, and developing the capacity to update patient images in near-real time as doctors practice their procedures.

When hardware costs are no longer a limiting factor, Stephanides believes VR technology will replace current surgical planning methods and become an important tool for educating doctors in medical schools.

Chapter 12

Endoscopic Plastic Surgery

If Your Doctor has Recommended Endoscopy

Endoscopy is a surgical technique that involves the use of an endoscope, a special viewing instrument that allows a surgeon to see images of the body's internal structures through very small incisions.

Endoscopic surgery has been used for decades in a number of different procedures, including gallbladder removal, tubal ligation, and knee surgery. However, in the world of plastic surgery, endoscopic instruments have recently been introduced. Plastic surgeons believe the technique holds great promise, but further study is needed to establish its effectiveness, especially over the long term. As important research continues, endoscopy is being used on a limited basis for both cosmetic and reconstructive procedures.

This text will give you a basic understanding of endoscopy in plastic surgery—how it's performed, what risks are involved, and the type of surgical training to look for in a surgeon. Please ask your doctor if there is anything you don't understand about the specific procedure you're planning to have.

The Endoscope

An endoscope consists of two basic parts: A tubular probe fitted with a tiny camera and bright light, which is inserted through a small incision; and a viewing screen, which magnifies the transmitted images of the body's internal structures. During surgery, the surgeon watches the screen while moving the tube of the endoscope through the surgical area.

It's important to understand that the endoscope functions as a viewing device only. To perform the surgery, a separate surgical instrument—such as a scalpel, scissors, or forceps—must be inserted through a different point of entry and manipulated within the tissue.

Advantages of Endoscopy

All surgery carries risks and every incision leaves a scar. However, with endoscopic surgery, your scars are likely to be hidden, much smaller and some of the after effects of surgery may be minimized.

In a typical endoscopic procedure, only a few small incisions, each less than one inch long, are needed to insert the endoscope probe and other instruments. For some procedures, such as breast augmentation, only two incisions may be necessary. For others, such as a forehead lift, three or more short incisions may be needed. The tiny "eye" of the endoscope's camera allows a surgeon to view the surgical site almost clearly as if the skin were opened from a long incision.

Because the incisions are shorter with endoscopy, the risk of sensory loss from nerve damage is decreased. Also, bleeding, bruising and swelling may be significantly reduced. With the endoscopic approach, you may recover more quickly and return to work earlier than if you had undergone open surgery.

Endoscopic surgery may also allow you to avoid an overnight hospital stay. Many endoscopic procedures can be performed on an outpatient basis under local anesthesia with sedation. Be sure to discuss this possibility with your doctor.

Uses in Plastic Surgery

As research continues, it's expected that many new uses for endoscopy will be developed. In the meantime, some plastic surgeons are using the technique on carefully selected patients. Some procedures that may be assisted by endoscopy are:

Cosmetic Surgery

Abdominoplasty (tummy tuck)—Endoscopy is sometimes used as an adjunct for selected patients who have lost abdominal muscle tone.

Guided by the endoscope, the muscles that run vertically down the length of the abdomen may be tightened through several short incisions. Endoscopy is generally not used in patients who have a significant amount of loose abdominal skin.

Breast augmentation—Inserted through a small incision in the underarm or the navel, an endoscope can assist the surgeon in positioning breast implants within the chest wall. Endoscopy may also assist in the correction of capsular contracture (scar tissue that sometimes forms around an implant, causing it to feel firm), and in the evaluation of existing implants.

Facelift—Although the traditional facelift operation is still the best choice for most patients—especially those with a significant amount of excess skin—certain selected individuals may benefit from an endoscopically assisted procedure. When an endoscope is used, the customary incision along, or in the hairline is usually eliminated. Instead, small incisions may be strategically placed in areas where the most correction is needed. If the muscles and skin of the mid-face need to be smoothed and tightened, incisions may be hidden in the lower eyelid and in the upper gumline. To tighten the loose muscles of the neck, incisions may be concealed beneath the chin and behind the ears. The endoscope may also assist in the positioning of cheek and chin implants.

Forehead lift—Of all the cosmetic procedures that use endoscopy, forehead lift is the one which plastic surgeons more commonly perform. Instead of the usual ear-to-ear incision, three or more "puncture-type" incisions are made just at the hairline. The endoscope helps guide the surgeon, who removes the muscles that produce frown lines, and repositions the eyebrows at a higher level.

Reconstructive Surgery

Flap surgery—Endoscopy can assist in repairing body parts that are damaged from injury or illness. Often, healthy tissue is "borrowed" from one part of the body to help repair another. Using an endoscope, the tissue or flaps can be removed from the donor site with only two or three small incisions.

Placement of tissue expanders—Used frequently in reconstructive surgery, tissue expanders are silicone "balloons" that are temporarily implanted to help stretch areas of healthy skin. The newly expanded skin is then used to cover body areas where skin has been lost due to injury (such as a burn) or disease. Using an endoscope, a surgeon can help ensure that a tissue expander is precisely positioned beneath the surface to bring the greatest benefit to the patient.

Sinus surgery—An endoscope can assist a surgeon in pinpointing and correcting sinus drainage problems. It can also help locate nasal polyps (growths) or other problems within the sinus cavity, and assist in full rhino-septal surgery.

Carpal tunnel release—After the endoscope is inserted through a small incision in the wrist area, the surgeon locates the median nerve, which runs down the center of the wrist. A separate incision may be made in the palm to insert scissors or scalpel to cut the ligament putting pressure on the nerve.

Finding a Well-Trained Surgeon

Because endoscopy is a relatively new technique in plastic surgery, it's extremely important that you select a board-certified plastic surgeon who has adequate training and experience.

Many endoscopic procedures do not require a hospital stay and are performed in a surgeon's office or an out-patient surgery center. If you're planning to have out-patient surgery, be sure that the surgeon you've selected has privileges to perform your particular endoscopic procedure at an accredited hospital. This assures you that your surgeon has been evaluated by the hospital's quality-assurance review committee and is generally considered to have the needed training.

Be sure to find out if the surgeon's hospital privileges cover both the endoscopic and the open version of the procedure you plan to have, since your doctor may have to switch to a traditional open procedure if a complication occurs during surgery.

Keep in mind that many plastic surgeons in practice today received endoscopy training as part of their plastic surgery or general surgery residency training. And, all board-certified plastic surgeons are continually being trained in new procedures.

Special Consideration and Risks

It's important to keep in mind that the endoscopic approach has only recently been applied to plastic surgery procedures. There are some known risks, which vary in severity depending on the procedure being performed. These include infection, fluid accumulation beneath the skin (which must be drained), blood vessel damage, nerve damage or loss of feeling, internal perforation injury, and skin injury.

And, keep in mind that if a complication occurs at any time during the operation your surgeon may have to switch to an open procedure, which will result in a more extensive scar and a longer recovery period. However, to date, such complications are rare—estimated to occur in less that 5 percent of all endoscopy procedures.

Deciding if Endoscopic Surgery is Right for You

Although much is still unknown about endoscopic plastic surgery, you may want to focus on what is known as you make your decision. Considering the following:

- For decades, endoscopy has been used successfully in orthopedic, urologic, and gynecologic procedures. Improved technology now permits endoscopy to be used by plastic surgeons.

- If performed by an experienced, well-trained plastic surgeon, endoscopic procedures may provide the same results as open-method procedures, but with less scarring.

- In some cases, endoscopic surgery may require less recovery time than is usually required for open procedures.

- Patients who tend to be the best candidates for cosmetic endoscopic procedures are those who don't have large amounts of loose hanging skin. Patients with loose facial or abdominal skin may benefit from a combination of classic and endoscopic techniques, in face or forehead lift, or abdominoplasty.

Additional information on plastic surgery is available from the Plastic Surgery Information Service web site at www.plasticsurgery.org or call (800) 635-0635.

Chapter 13

Ultrasound-Assisted Lipoplasty

If You're Considering UAL

Ultrasound-assisted lipoplasty, commonly known as "UAL," is a relatively new liposuction technique that uses sound waves to "liquefy" unwanted fat. Although it is not a substitute for traditional liposuction, UAL can be an effective tool for removing fat from fibrous body areas, such as the male breasts or the back, or for removing larger volumes of fat in a single procedure.

Often, traditional liposuction is performed with UAL to help shape UAL-treated areas or to treat areas of the body not suited for UAL, such as the neck and inner thighs.

If you are considering UAL, this information will provide an overview of the technique: when it can help, how it is performed and what results you can expect. It can't answer all of your questions, since a lot depends on your individual circumstances. Ultimately, you and your plastic surgeon will determine whether UAL or traditional liposuction is best suited for you.

Please ask your physician if there is anything about the procedure you don't understand.

The Best Candidates for UAL

Liposuction can enhance your appearance and your self confidence, but it won't necessarily change your looks to match your ideal, or cause

Southern California Plastic Surgery Group, reprinted from. http://www.face-doctor.com. © 1994; reprinted with permission.

71

other people to treat you differently. Before you decide to have UAL or liposuction of any type, think carefully about your expectations and discuss them with your surgeon.

The best candidates for UAL are generally no different than candidates for the traditional liposuction procedure: normal-weight people with firm, elastic skin who have pockets of excess fat in particular areas. UAL candidates should be physically healthy, psychologically stable and realistic in their expectations. Age is usually not a criterion for liposuction, but older patients may have diminished skin elasticity and may not achieve the same results as a younger patient.

All surgery carries some uncertainty and risk. Since it was first described in the medical literature in 1991, UAL has been performed on several thousand patients worldwide. However, long-term effects of ultrasound energy are not known and extensive research and clinical trials are needed to establish fully the safety and efficacy of UAL. So far, clinical investigators have reported good results from the technique.

UAL is normally safe when patients are carefully selected, the operating facility is properly equipped and the physician has completed an appropriate, hands-on UAL training course.

As with traditional liposuction, serious medical complications from UAL are infrequent. However, possible complications include clots that block blood flow, infection, excessive fluid loss that can lead to shock, excessive fluid accumulation that must be drained, skin injury, perforation injury to the skin or other organs and adverse reactions to anesthesia.

One potential complication specifically related to the UAL technique is thermal skin injury or burn caused by the heat from the ultrasound device. Also, temporary collections of fluid beneath the skin surface (seromas) are more common with UAL.

Also, you should be aware that at present, the tube-like instruments or cannulas used to perform UAL are slightly larger than the cannulas used for traditional liposuction. The longer incisions that are needed for UAL require that they be placed carefully in hidden areas. For this reason, some surgeons prefer to use the traditional liposuction technique in areas where an obvious scar may result.

Cosmetic complications from all types of liposuction include: irregularities of the skin's surface, areas of uneven pigmentation, and asymmetry. Some cosmetic problems can be treated with additional surgery.

Planning Your Surgery

In your initial consultation, your surgeon will evaluate your health, determine where your fat deposits lie and assess the condition of your skin. Your surgeon will explain the body contouring methods that may be most appropriate for you. For example, you may learn that an abdominoplasty or "tummy tuck" may more effectively meet your goals; or that a combination of traditional liposuction and UAL would be the best choice for you.

Be frank in discussing your expectations with your surgeon. Also, be sure to tell your physician about any significant weight losses or gains you have had at any time. You should inform your surgeon if you smoke, and if you're taking any medications, vitamins or other drugs.

Preparing for Your Surgery

Your surgeon will give you specific instructions on how to prepare for surgery, including guidelines on eating and drinking, smoking, and taking or avoiding vitamins, iron tablets and certain medications. If you develop a cold or an infection of any kind, especially a skin infection, your procedure may have to be postponed.

While you are making preparations, be sure to arrange for someone to drive you home after your surgery and, if needed, to help you out for a day or two.

Where Your Surgery Will Be Performed

UAL may be performed in a surgeon's office-based facility, an outpatient surgery center, or a hospital. It is usually done on an outpatient basis. If a large volume of fat will be removed, a stay in a hospital or overnight nursing facility may be required.

Anesthesia for UAL

If you are having only a small amount of fat removed, UAL may be performed under local anesthesia combined with a sedative to make you drowsy. You will be awake but relaxed and feel only minimal discomfort. Some surgeons may prefer to use an epidural block, similar to the anesthesia commonly used in childbirth. General anesthesia may be used if you prefer it, or if your doctor so advises. In that case, you will sleep through the procedure.

The Surgery

The time required to perform UAL may vary considerably, depending on the amount of work you are having done. However, UAL generally takes longer than traditional liposuction because of the extra "fat-liquefying" step involved.

To begin the procedure, salt water containing local anesthesia and adrenaline is injected into the area to be treated. Then, a metal cannula connected to an ultrasound generator is inserted beneath the skin through a small incision. The ultrasonic energy causes the walls of the fat cells to break down, allowing the fat to flow out of each cell. The "liquefied" fat combines with the injected fluid to create an emulsion, which is removed from the body by vacuum pressure.

If you are awake, you may feel some warmth and vibration during the procedure. You will probably be given some fluid through an IV (intravenous) tube to keep your fluid level balanced. Typically, only a small amount of blood is lost during UAL. However, if your surgeon determines that a blood transfusion may be needed, you can donate your own blood in advance of the procedure.

After Your Surgery

After surgery, you will likely experience some fluid drainage from the incisions. A drainage tube may be inserted beneath the skin to prevent fluid build-up. To help control swelling, you may be fitted with a snug elastic bandage or compression garment to wear over the treated area. The bandage or garment is typically worn for up to four weeks, to help your skin shrink to fit its new contour.

The side-effects of traditional liposuction surgery—pain, burning, swelling, bleeding, and temporary numbness—can be expected from UAL as well. The pain can be controlled with medications prescribed by your surgeon, though you may still feel stiff and sore for a few days.

It is normal to feel a bit depressed in the days or weeks following surgery. This feeling will subside as you begin to look and feel better.

Getting Back to Normal

Healing is a gradual process. Your surgeon will probably tell you to start walking around as soon as possible. You will begin to feel better after about a week and you should be back to work within two weeks following your surgery. Any stitches are usually removed within the first week.

Activity that is more strenuous should be avoided for about three weeks as your body continues to heal. Although most of the bruising and swelling usually disappears within six weeks, some swelling may remain for six months or more.

Your surgeon will schedule follow-up visits to monitor your progress and to see if any additional procedures are needed.

Your New Look

You will see a noticeable difference in the shape of your body quite soon after surgery. However, improvement will become even more apparent after about six weeks, when most of the swelling has subsided.

If your expectations are realistic, you will probably be very pleased with the results of your surgery. You may find that you are more comfortable in a wide variety of clothes and more at ease with your body. And, by eating a healthy diet and getting regular exercise, you can help to maintain your new shape permanently.

Chapter 14

New Breast Reduction Technique May Offer Longer-Lasting Results, Less Scarring

A new method of breast reduction that combines decreased scarring with the safety and familiarity of traditional methods has obtained better surgical results, according to a new study in the March issue of the journal *Plastic and Reconstructive Surgery*.

To date, the most common breast reduction procedure results in a wide, inverted T-scar. While this procedure has a successful proven history, loss of breast contour or bottoming out can occur. The long scar running under the breast can also be undesirable.

Alternative short-scar techniques have been developed using the superior pedicle (tissue situated on the top part of the breast through which blood is supplied to the nipple and areola). However, these techniques are not widely applied as many surgeons are either unfamiliar with the superior pedicle or believe it to be less reliable. Moving the nipple and areola with this method may restrict the blood supply to these areas. Predicting ultimate nipple and areola position on the breast is also more difficult. Relying heavily on postoperative settling for final breast shape further limits control over results.

This latest method, as detailed in the study, builds upon the best aspects of the previous techniques. It is a short scar procedure that uses the preferred, traditional inferior pedicle (tissue situated on the bottom part of the breast) and offers consistent, controllable results over breast shape.

"By combining the aesthetic advantage of less cutaneous scarring with the safety and familiarity of the inferiorly based pedicle, superior results in breast reduction can be obtained that are consistent, long-lasting and satisfying for both patient and surgeon alike," said Dennis Hammond, M.D., a Grand Rapids, Michigan, an American Society of Plastic and Reconstructive Surgeons (ASPRS) member and author of the study. "By retaining fat and parenchyma (the main tissue of the breast) centrally beneath the nipple and areola, direct contouring of the breast with consistent control over shape becomes possible. Very little reliance is placed on postoperative settling, with essentially no bottoming out."

The study was conducted with 98 women. Patients with six months of follow-up were graded for scar quality. Of these patients, 83 percent were graded as having fine line to slightly spread scars around the areola, with 17 percent having widened scars. Skin wrinkling around the areola was absent or minimal in 89 percent, mild in eight percent and marked in three percent.

Delayed wound healing developed in 13 percent of patients and was successfully treated with topical agents. Fat necrosis (cell death) developed in eight patients, and partial areola necrosis developed in six breasts (four patients). Only two patients in the study showed any extension of the lower breast contour below the postoperative inframammary fold. Only one patient ultimately required scar revision. There were no cases of nipple and areola complex loss, infection or hematoma in the study.

Chapter 15

New Grafting Material Improves Defects Over Time

Autologous fibroblast grafting may be the only approach for filling dermal defects that actually improves results over time, Dr. Victor LaCombe said at a meeting sponsored by the American Academy of Facial Plastic and Reconstructive Surgery (ASPRS). This approach may be useful for correcting glabellar furrows, periorbital rhytids, acne scars, and other defects. Autologous collagen or fat, porcine collagen, silicone, and most other grafting materials are all absorbed or broken down to varying degrees over time, resulting in a gradual diminution of the cosmetic result in the months or years following injection.

Autologous fibroblasts, which are grown from a small punch biopsy sample of the patient's own skin, are self-perpetuating and continue to generate new collagen—resulting in ever-greater filling of the defect over the course of time, explained Dr. LaCombe of the division of head and neck surgery at the University of California, Los Angeles.

Dr. LaCombe and his colleague, Dr. Gregory Keller, are among 40 clinical research teams currently studying autologous fibroblast grafting for cosmetic surgical applications. Dr. Keller, who has used the technique in approximately 350 patients, described the results as cosmetically excellent, with no infections or inflammation and high patient satisfaction.

"New Grafting Material Improves Defects Over Time: Autologous Fibroblasts are Self-Perpetuating and Continue to Generate New Collagen," by Erik L. Goldman, New York Bureau, in *Skin & Allergy News,* Vol. 30, No. (5), pgs. 1,4. © 1999 International Medical News Group; reprinted with permission.

The UCLA team uses fibroblast cell lines prepared from patients' postauricular skin samples by a company called Isolagen, located in Paramus, N.J. Between six and seven weeks after a tissue sample is sent, Isolagen returns—via overnight delivery—premeasured 3-cc syringes with 30-gauge needles containing the patient's own fibroblasts suspended in a special medium. Each defect usually requires three injections. Isolagen recommends allowing two-week intervals between injection sessions. Isolagen, explained Dr. Keller, has a patent on this particular packaging of fibroblast technology for cosmetic application. Other companies and research laboratories across the country also are growing fibroblast cell lines for a range of different clinical applications.

In a small study of 10 patients, the UCLA researchers used the Isolagen grafts to treat glabellar lines, periorbital rhytids, nasolabial creases, and depressed acne scars. To measure improvement, they took preoperative photos and silicone molds of the defects, which could be assessed via optical profilometry. They repeated their assessments every two to three months for a total of 24 months.

The results were highly consistent. By the third month, there was significant graft persistence, marked reduction of defect depth, and good patient satisfaction. "By six months, the improvement was even better. The injected cells continue growing and laying down dermal collagen. You get more improvement, not less," said Dr. LaCombe. At 24 months, there were no adverse effects and no evidence of resorption or reversal of the correction. Dr. LaCombe noted that results tend to be best in younger patients.

Dr. Keller added that this technique is especially good for correcting acne scars. "We don't recommend it for crow's feet or active muscle defects."

There are three main drawbacks to Isolagen injections: pain, cost, and timing. Dr. LaCombe noted that this technique tends to be more painful than collagen injections, warranting the use of EMLA and in some cases dental nerve blocking techniques.

Autologous fibroblast injection is expensive. Dr. Keller told this newspaper that Isolagen charges approximately $500 per syringe. "We sell the patients packages of three injections. One usually will not do it." He noted that his clinic charges patients $3,500 per series of three injections. Timing of the injections is critical. "You must inject on the day (the fibroblast-filled syringes) are received," said Dr. LaCombe. This means the patient must be extremely diligent in showing up for the scheduled appointments. The fibroblast cultures are extremely fragile and will die unless immediately injected. Dr. Keller noted that for a fee the Isolagen company will store a patient's fibroblast culture for later regrowth. If properly handled, they can be kept indefinitely.

Cultured fibroblasts as prepared by Isolagen are in limbo regulation wise, said Robert Mazurek, Isolagen's executive vice president of sales and marketing. Mr. Mazurek told this newspaper that Food and Drug Administration officials are currently reviewing the existing data on the fibroblast culture technique. He expects the FDA to make a determination sometime this spring as to how this "minimally manipulated biological" will be regulated and whether further research is needed. Until the regulations are fully defined, Isolagen will not accept new patient biopsies. The company will continue to produce fibroblast grafts for clinicians already engaged in research protocols, Mr. Mazurek said. Dr. LaCombe and Dr. Keller said that they had no financial ties to Isolagen.

Chapter 16

Technique Enhances Hand Surgery Results

Fine strands of fatty tissue, interwoven like a basket, can better restore atrophied subcutaneous tissue on the back of the hand, for a more youthful and healthy appearance, according to a study that was to be presented at the annual meeting of the American Association for Hand Surgery in Honolulu last month [January 1999].

Structural fat transplantation, in which large amounts of fat are injected subcutaneously, has been used since 1991 mainly for cosmetic purposes. Sydney R. Coleman, M.D., a plastic surgeon in private practice in New York, has refined this technique. He makes more injections, but each contains only tiny amounts of fat. As many as 10 or 20 passes are used to inject 1 cc of fat. "Think of it like pearls on a string," Dr. Coleman said. "You put in tiny threads and interweave them like a basket. Putting in the fat in miniscule portions gives it a chance to anchor." When fat is inserted in larger amounts, it tends to form lumps, and as much as 50 percent of it may not survive the operation, he explained.

The fat used in the transplantation technique is harvested from another part of the patient's body, generally the abdomen or thigh, by liposuction using a 10 cc syringe attached to a 2 mm cannula, Dr. Coleman explained. The fat is removed slowly, without exposure to air and without negative or positive pressure. The fat is then purified

"Technique Enhances Hand Surgery Results: Refinement of Existing Procedure Involves Injection of Tiny Amounts of Fat Subcutaneously," by Ann Saul, from meeting coverage of the American Association for Hand Surgery, February 4, 1999. © 1999 Medical Tribune; reprinted with permission.

in a centrifuge, which separates it from the oil, water and lidocaine that are also present in the extracted substance.

To perform the procedure, five 1 mm incisions are made on the back of the hand, two at the wrist and three at the bases of the first, second and fourth web spaces, Dr. Coleman explained. Using an 18-gauge blunt cannula, fine strands of fat are carefully placed in the subcutaneous layers from the wrist to the interphalangeal joints of the index through the small fingers and to the interphalangeal joint of the thumb. The entire surgical procedure requires about two hours, he said. "The skin is like chiffon, and we're putting a silk backing on it," explained Dr. Coleman, who has performed this procedure on 50 women and two men who suffered from loss of subcutaneous tissue due to aging, steroid administration, prominent veins and tendons, and intermetacarpal wasting.

The scaffolding or weaving of the fatty tissue provides additional support for the skin on the back of the hand, giving it a more youthful appearance, masking intermetacarpal wasting, decreasing the visibility of prominent veins and tendons, and giving the skin improved color and texture.

Complications, such as subcutaneous irregularities, are dependent on the way the technique is performed, and the main side effect is mild swelling, according to David H. Ostad, M.D., a resident in plastic surgery at St. Luke's Roosevelt Hospital Center in New York. "This technique not only restores the subcutaneous tissue, but it makes the skin actually appear thicker. When a patient has cosmetic surgery on the face, his or her hand doesn't fit and that can give away the patient's age. This is another avenue for the patient," he said.

Part Four

Cosmetic Plastic Surgery

Chapter 17

Injectable Fillers: Improving Skin Texture

If You're Considering Injectables...

As we age, our faces begin to show the effects of gravity, sun exposure and years of facial muscle movement, such as smiling, chewing and squinting. The underlying tissues that keep our skin looking youthful and plumped up begin to break down, often leaving laugh lines, smile lines, crow's feet, or facial creases over the areas where this muscle movement occurs.

Soft-tissue fillers, most commonly injectable collagen or fat, can help fill in these lines and creases, temporarily restoring a smoother, more youthful-looking appearance. When injected beneath the skin, these fillers plump up creased and sunken areas of the face. They can also add fullness to the lips and cheeks. Injectable fillers may be used alone or in conjunction with a resurfacing procedure, such as a laser treatment, or a recontouring procedure, such as a facelift.

If you're considering a facial-rejuvenation treatment with collagen or fat, this chapter will give you a basic understanding of the procedure—when injectables can help, how the procedure is performed, and what results you can expect. It may not answer all of your questions, since a lot depends on your individual circumstances. Please ask your doctor if there is anything about the procedure you don't understand.

Southern California Plastic Surgery Group, reprinted from. http://www.face-doctor.com. © 1994; reprinted with permission.

Knowing Your Options

Injectables are usually not sufficient for severe surface wrinkles on the face, such as multiple vertical "lipstick lines" that sometimes form around the mouth. Instead, your plastic surgeon may suggest a resurfacing technique, such as chemical peel, dermabrasion or laser treatments. Rather than filling in facial lines, resurfacing methods strip away the outer layers of the skin to produce a smoother appearance.

Deep folds in the face or brow caused by overactive muscles or by loose skin may be more effectively treated with cosmetic surgery, such as a facelift or browlift. Injectables are sometimes used in conjunction with facial surgery procedures, however, injectables alone cannot change facial contour the way surgery can.

Keep in mind that a plastic surgeon is a specialist that can offer you the full gamut of the most advanced treatments ranging from cosmetic surgery, refinishing techniques, laser therapy, injectables and the use of other fillers. You and your surgeon may determine that a single procedure or a combination of procedures is the best choice for you. The American Society of Plastic Surgeons (ASPS) brochures are available on chemical peel, dermabrasion, laser treatments, facelift, and browlift. If you and your doctor think that one of these other procedures might be more appropriate for you, ask your plastic surgeon to provide you with a copy.

Injectable collagen or fat can help improve the skin's texture by filling in the laugh lines and facial creases that often occur with aging.

A Word about Other Types of Fillers

This chapter deals with the two most commonly used types of injectable fillers: collagen and fat. However, to a lesser extent, a number of other filler materials are also being used for facial-rejuvenation purposes. They include: Fibril, a gelatin powder compound that's mixed with a patient's own blood and is injected to plump up the skin (similar to injectable collagen); and Gortex, a thread-like material that is implanted beneath the skin to add soft-tissue support. Each of these options has its own set of risks and benefits. If you're considering any of these alternative filler treatments, tell your doctor.

What to Expect from Treatment

The most important fact to remember about injectable fillers is that the results are not permanent. Injected material is eventually metabolized by the body. You should not expect the same long-lasting results that may be gained from cosmetic surgery.

In some individuals, the results may last only a few weeks; in others, the results may be maintained indefinitely. Researchers believe that age, genetic background, skin quality and lifestyle as well as the injected body site may all play a role in the injected material's "staying power." However, the precise reason for the variation of results among patients has yet to be identified.

If you've had short-lived results from fat injections, you shouldn't necessarily assume that collagen injections will work better for you. And, conversely, if you've had disappointing results from collagen, don't assume that injected fat is the answer. Although it's true that some individuals' bodies are more receptive to one substance than the other, others may find that neither substance produces long-lasting results. Sometimes one substance may work better than the other for a specific problem.

Risks Related to Injectables

When injectables are administered by a qualified plastic surgeon, complications are infrequent and usually minor in nature. Still, individuals vary greatly in their anatomy, their physical reactions and their healing abilities. The outcome of treatment with injectables is never completely predictable.

Collagen: Allergic reaction is the primary risk of collagen. To help determine if you are allergic to the substance, your surgeon will perform an allergy skin test about a month before the procedure. After the test is performed, the test site should be watched carefully for three or four weeks, or as long as your surgeon advises. Any sign of redness, itching, swelling or other occurrences at the test site should be reported to your surgeon.

Risks not necessarily related to allergies include infection, abscesses, open sores, skin peeling, scarring, and lumpiness, which may persist over the treated area. Reports of these problems are very rare.

Fat: Allergic reaction is not a factor for fat because it's harvested from a patient's own body. However, there is still a small risk of infection and other infrequent complications.

Planning for Treatment

Facial rejuvenation is very individualized. That's why it's important to discuss your hopes and expectations with a board-certified plastic surgeon who has experience with many different types of surgical and non-surgical facial procedures.

In your initial consultation, your plastic surgeon will evaluate your face—the skin, the muscles and the underlying bone—and discuss your goals for the surgery. Your doctor will help you select a treatment option based on your goals and concerns, your anatomy and your lifestyle.

Your surgeon will ask you about your medical history, drug allergies, and check for conditions that could cause problems, such as active skin infections or non-healed sores from injuries. Collagen injections are generally off limits for pregnant women, individuals who are allergic to beef or bovine products, patients who suffer from autoimmune diseases, and those who are allergic to lidocaine (the anesthetic agent contained in the syringe with the collagen material). For more specific information about the contraindications and risks of collagen use, ask your doctor for the manufacturer's brochure for patients.

Insurance usually doesn't cover cosmetic procedures. However, if your injectable treatment is being performed to treat a scar or indentation from an accident or injury, you may be reimbursed for a portion of the cost. Check with your insurance carrier to be sure.

Where Your Treatment Will Be Performed

Injectables are usually administered in a surgeon's office-based facility. If, however, you are being hospitalized for a facelift, necklift, browlift, or any other procedure, your injections may be administered in the hospital as well.

Types of Anesthesia

Collagen: Because the anesthetic agent lidocaine is mixed in with collagen, additional anesthetic is usually not used. However, if you are especially sensitive to pain, your doctor may use a topical cream anesthetic or a freon spray to numb the injected area. Or, you may elect to have an injected local anesthetic or sedative drugs.

Fat: Both the donor and recipient sites are numbed with local anesthesia. Sedation can be used as well. If you elect to use sedation, be sure to arrange for a ride home after your treatment.

The Treatments

Collagen

Collagen is a naturally occurring protein that provides support to various parts of the human body: the skin, the joints, the bones and the ligaments. Injectable collagen, patented by the Collagen Corporation under the trade names Zyderm and Zyplast, is derived from purified bovine collagen. The purification process creates a product similar to human collagen. Injectable collagen received approval from the Food and Drug Administration in 1981. It is produced in various thicknesses to meet individual patient needs.

Collagen is used primarily to fill wrinkles, lines and scars on the face and sometimes the neck, back and chest.

The procedure: Treatment with collagen can begin after a skin test determines that you're not allergic to the substance. The collagen is injected using a fine needle inserted at several points along the edge of the treatment site. If a local anesthesia has not been used, you may feel some minor stinging or burning as the injections are administered.

Since part of the substance is salt water that will be absorbed by the body within a few days, your doctor will slightly overfill the area. You may be asked to hold a hand mirror during the procedure to help your doctor decide when you've had enough.

After treatment: Immediately following treatment, you may notice some minor discomfort, stinging or throbbing in the injected area. Occasionally some bruising or swelling will occur, but it is usually minor. Any redness that appears in the injected site usually disappears within 24 hours. However, in some individuals, particularly fair-skinned patients, this redness may persist for a week or more. Tiny scabs may also form over the needle-stick areas; these generally heal quickly.

No bandaging is needed and you are free to eat, drink, and wear makeup with sunblock protection shortly thereafter. There may be some temporary swelling and redness in the treated area which should dissipate within a few days. If these symptoms persist, contact your surgeon.

Results: As stated earlier, the duration of results from collagen injections is variable. Collagen's longevity depends on the patient's lifestyle and physical characteristics as well as the part of the body treated. In general, the injected material is likely to disappear faster in areas that are more affected by muscle movement.

Your doctor can help you determine how long you can go between treatments to best maintain your results.

Fat

In the medical world, the fat-injection procedure is known as autologous fat transplantation or microlipoinjection. It involves extracting fat cells from the patient's abdomen, thighs, buttocks or elsewhere and reinjecting them beneath the facial skin. Fat is most often used to fill in "sunken" cheeks or laugh lines between the nose and mouth, to correct skin depressions or indentations, to minimize forehead wrinkles and to enhance the lips.

The procedure: After both the donor and recipient sites are cleansed and treated with a local anesthesia, the fat is withdrawn using a syringe with a large-bore needle or a cannula (the same instrument used in liposuction) attached to a suction device. The fat is then prepared and injected into the recipient site with a needle. Sometimes an adhesive bandage is applied over the injection site.

As with collagen, "overfilling" is necessary to allow for fat absorption in the weeks following treatment. When fat is used to fill sunken cheeks or to correct areas on the face other than lines, this over-correction of newly injected fat may temporarily make the face appear abnormally puffed out or swollen.

After treatment: If a larger area was treated, you may be advised to curtail your activity for a brief time. However, many patients are able to resume normal activity immediately. You can expect some swelling, bruising or redness in both the donor and recipient sites. The severity of these symptoms depends upon the size and location of the treated area. You should stay out of the sun until the redness and bruising subsides—usually about 48 hours. In the meantime, you may use makeup with sunblock protection to help conceal your condition.

The swelling and puffiness in the recipient site may last several weeks, especially if a large area was filled.

Results: The duration of the fat injections varies significantly from patient to patient. Though some patients have reported results lasting a year or more, the majority of patients find that at least half of the injected fullness disappears within 3-6 months. Therefore, repeated injections may be necessary. Your doctor will advise you on how to maintain your results with repeat treatments.

Your New Look

If you're like most patients, you'll be very satisfied with the results of your injectable treatments. You may be surprised at the pleasing results that can be gained from this procedure.

Chapter 18

Face-Lift:
The Traditional Operation

A face-lift is an operation that elevates and re-drapes the facial skin and muscles to eliminate laxity and sagging. The operation can be designed to correct problems in the neck, under the jaw, under the chin and in the cheeks. It can also be applied to the skin in the temporal regions and the forehead.

As individuals age, there is a change in the skin just as there are changes in all other parts of the body. Fatty tissue tends to decrease in volume and in density causing the skin to fit more loosely. There are also changes in the bones of the face, which combine with changes in muscular action and gravity leading to more prominent skin folds. These changes are greatest under the chin, in the upper neck and at the skin folds near the corner of the mouth. Contour imperfections of the nose may also become more noticeable as the overlying soft tissue decreases in volume.

The traditional face-lift operation is designed to improve these facial conditions. A general anesthetic is usually selected although the surgery can be performed under local anesthesia with sedation. The operation involves lifting and removing the excess skin. However, an equally important part is the tightening and support of the underlying tissues and muscle, which helps to give a longer lasting result.

Another important aspect of the operation is the removal of the excess fatty tissue found in the neck and jowls of many patients. This

Howard A. Tobin, M.D., F.A.C.S., Facial Plastic & Cosmetic Surgical Center, reprinted from the website at www.newlook.com. © 2000; reprinted with permission.

is usually removed with micro-liposuction surgery which has become a standard part of the modern face-lift operation. For additional details about liposuction surgery, please prefer to that chapter in this book.

The incisions for a facelift will vary depending on the exact problem to be corrected, but usually involve an incision extending from the temple, wrapping around the ear and ending in the hair behind the ear. We have developed a "hair sparing" technique" in which we advance tissue rather than excise it in hair bearing areas. The major pull of the operation is on deeper structures rather than skin. This means that little or no hair is removed during surgery. In all cases, the incisions are placed in areas where they will be well hidden. In exposed areas, very fine absorbable suture is used which is nearly invisible from the start. Consideration will be given to whether the patient is male or female, hair pattern, areas that need most correction, etc. This is reviewed individually with each patient.

Surgical treatment of facial sagging will result in limited benefit where very fine skin wrinkles are the most prominent deformity. There are other means to achieve improvement of these surface conditions such as laser treatment or chemical peel. In many cases, regional surface treatment can be combined with face lifting. We have found that by combining laser resurfacing with a facelift, the benefits of both are enhanced. Surface surgery, including laser, is covered in a separate chapter in this book.

There has been a large increase in the popularity of the face-lift operation as a result of the improvements in techniques. Patients are now seeking surgery at an earlier age. There is no upper and lower age limit for the operation. While correction is perfectly possible in the late sixties or early seventies, over stretched muscles with lack of tone become more difficult to repair, and the result, while still good, may not be as long-lasting. When surgery is carried out at a younger age, the results certainly last longer, although the initial change will not be as striking. Indeed, patients in their thirties have face-lifts with very satisfactory results.

Forehead and Brow Lift

The standard face-lift is most effective in improving the mid and lower face, as well as the neck. Additional procedures, which can be done either with the standard face-lift, or as separate operations, help to improve the forehead, temple and brow regions.

Secondary Face-Lift

The results of a face-lift can be lasting. Although the procedure does not stop the aging process, it certainly slows down the clock. An individual who has a face-lift will probably always look younger than he or she would have, had the operation not been performed. Furthermore, a secondary face-lift (a much less extensive procedure) carried out a year or so after the initial operation appears to produce a much more lasting effect. This is because the original operation results in a network of thin scar tissue beneath the skin. The scar tissue is "stiffer" than normal subcutaneous tissue and holds better when tightened. This so-called secondary tuck has become very popular among patients who have had a facelift. The recovery from this secondary operation is prompt with many patients resuming normal activity within a day or so. Because there is much less dissection involved, this surgery can be carried out under local or light general anesthesia.

Of equal importance is the fact that secondary lifts carried out after a complete face-lift is much less expensive than the original surgery. For some patients, it is considered maintenance treatment.

Risks and Complications

Complications are relatively infrequent in a well performed facelift. There can be some blood collection under the skin—a condition called hematoma. This is much more common in men and especially in smokers. This often can be treated during the follow-up office examination and will not affect the overall results.

Larger collections may require earlier and more vigorous treatment and could possibly require reopening of the surgical incision to remove the clotted blood. Although post-operative bleeding usually will not prevent a satisfactory result from surgery, it can significantly delay complete recovery. For that reason, patients must understand that recovery times that are discussed are estimates that can vary considerably.

There may be some temporary lag in the normal motion of the facial muscles. Generally this is related to the local anesthetic that is used to supplement the general anesthetic. In rare cases, this weakness could be longer lasting and perhaps even permanent.

Scarring is a natural sequel of any incision. Some people heal with better scars than others. Because of their placement, facelift scars are hardly noticeable. If they are a problem, they can often be improved by injections of a scar softener or a minor secondary scar revision. Scars always look worst shortly after surgery, and it takes a full year for them to fade to their best appearance.

While infection is rare after facelift surgery, as with all operations, it is possible, and while usually readily amenable to antibiotic treatment, it can on occasion be serious or difficult to treat.

Recovery from the Facelift Operation

Dressings are generally not used by us after facelift surgery. We find that patients are more comfortable without them. Additionally, if problems develop, dressings may hide them and make them more difficult to diagnose. Patients wear an elastic neck strap part time for a few weeks after surgery. Initially there may be a feeling of numbness and tension in the operative area. This usually disappears within the first few weeks but may last longer. Swelling and bruising vary but are usually gone within two weeks or so. Patients are active within a few days of surgery. Often there is a sense of tightness, which can last for several weeks or even months. Excessive turning of the neck is discouraged during this time. Make-up can be applied within a couple of days of surgery. It must be recognized that marked degrees of skin laxity may not be entirely correctable with one operation. Some recurrent sagging can take place even after the first few months. Minor secondary procedures might therefore be desirable to achieve maximum benefit.

For additional information contact: Howard A. Tobin, M.D., F.A.C.S., Facial Plastic & Cosmetic Surgical Center, 6300 Regional Plaza, Abilene, Texas 79606. (915) 695-3630; Toll Free (800) 592-4533; Fax (915) 695-3633; e-mail: n41gt@newlook.com.

Chapter 19

Forehead Lift (Including Endoscopy)

If You're Considering a Forehead Lift

A forehead lift or "browlift" is a procedure that restores a more youthful, refreshed look to the area above the eyes. The procedure corrects drooping brows and improves the horizontal lines and furrows that can make a person appear angry, sad or tired.

In a forehead lift, the muscles and tissues that cause the furrowing or drooping are removed or altered to smooth the forehead, raise the eyebrows and minimize frown lines. Your surgeon may use the conventional surgical method, in which the incision is hidden just behind the hairline; or it may be performed with the use of an endoscope, a viewing instrument that allows the procedure to be performed with minimal incisions. Both techniques yield similar results—smoother forehead skin and a more animated appearance.

If you're considering a forehead lift, this text will provide a basic understanding of the procedure—when it can help, how it's performed and what results you can expect. It won't answer all of your questions, since a lot depends on your individual circumstances. Be sure to ask your doctor if there is anything you don't understand about the procedure.

American Society of Plastic Surgeons, reprinted from The Plastic Surgery Information Service at www.plasticsurgery.org. © 1997; reprinted with permission.

The Best Candidates for a Forehead Lift

A forehead lift is most commonly performed in the 40-60 age range to minimize the visible effects of aging. However, it can also help people of any age who have developed furrows or frown lines due to stress or muscle activity. Individuals with inherited conditions, such as a low, heavy brow or furrowed lines above the nose can achieve a more alert and refreshed look with this procedure.

Forehead lift is often performed in conjunction with a facelift to provide a smoother overall look to the face. Eyelid surgery (blepharoplasty) may also be performed at the same time as a forehead lift, especially if a patient has significant skin overhang in the upper eyelids. Sometimes, patients who believe they need upper-eyelid surgery find that a forehead lift better meets their surgical goals.

Patients who are bald, who have a receding hairline, or who have had previous upper-eyelid surgery may still be good candidates for forehead lift. The surgeon will simply alter the incision location or perform a more conservative operation.

Remember, a forehead lift can enhance your appearance and your self-confidence, but it won't necessarily change your looks to match your ideal or cause other people to treat you differently. Before you decide to have surgery, think carefully about your expectations and discuss them in detail with your doctor.

All Surgery Carries Some Uncertainty and Risk

Complications are rare and usually minor when a forehead lift is performed by a qualified plastic surgeon. Yet, the possibility of complications must be considered. In rare cases, the nerves that control eyebrow movement may be injured on one or both sides, resulting in a loss of ability to raise the eyebrows or wrinkle the forehead. Additional surgery may be required to correct the problem.

Formation of a broad scar is also a rare complication. This may be treated surgically by removing the wide scar tissue so a new, thinner scar may result. Also, in some patients, hair loss may occur along the scar edges.

Loss of sensation along or just beyond the incision line is common, especially with the classic forehead lift procedure. It is usually temporary, but may be permanent in some patients. Infection and bleeding are very rare, but are possibilities.

If a complication should occur during an endoscopic forehead lift, your surgeon may have to abandon the endoscopic approach and switch to the conventional, open procedure, which will result in a more extensive scar and a longer recovery period. To date, such complications are rare—estimated at less than 1 percent of all endoscopy procedures.

You can reduce your risk of complications by closely following your surgeon's instructions both before and after surgery.

Planning Your Surgery

For a better understanding of how a forehead lift might change your appearance, look into a mirror and place the palms of your hands at the outer edges of your eyes, above your eyebrows. Gently draw the skin up to raise the brow and the forehead area. That is approximately what a forehead lift would do for you.

If you decide to consult a plastic surgeon, he or she will first evaluate your face, including the skin and underlying bone. During your consultation, the surgeon will discuss your goals for the surgery and ask you about certain medical conditions that could cause problems during or after the procedure, such as uncontrolled high blood pressure, blood-clotting problems, or the tendency to develop large scars. Be sure to tell the surgeon if you have had previous facial surgery, if you smoke, or if you take any drugs or medications—including aspirin or other drugs that affect clotting.

If you decide to proceed with a forehead lift, your surgeon will explain the surgical technique, the recommended type of anesthesia, the type of facility where the surgery will be performed, the risks and the costs involved. Don't hesitate to ask your doctor any questions you may have, especially those regarding your expectations and concerns about the results of surgery.

Preparing for Your Surgery

Your surgeon will give you specific instructions to prepare for the procedure, including guidelines on eating and drinking, smoking, and taking and avoiding certain vitamins and medications. Carefully following these instructions will help your surgery and your recovery proceed more smoothly.

If your hair is very short, you may wish to let it grow out before surgery, so that it's long enough to hide the scars while they heal. Whether your forehead lift is done in an outpatient facility or in the hospital, you should arrange for someone to drive you home after your surgery, and to help you out for a day or two.

Where Your Surgery Will Be Performed

A forehead lift is usually done in a surgeon's office-based facility or an outpatient surgery center. However, it is occasionally done in the hospital.

Anesthesia Used for the Procedure

Most forehead lifts are performed under local anesthesia, combined with a sedative to make you drowsy. You'll be awake but relaxed, and although you may feel some tugging and mild discomfort, your forehead will be insensitive to pain. Some surgeons prefer to use general anesthesia, in which case you'll sleep through the entire operation.

The Surgery

Your surgeon will help you decide which surgical approach will best achieve your cosmetic goals: the classic or "open" method, or the endoscopic forehead lift. Make sure you understand the technique that your surgeon recommends and why he or she feels it is best for you.

The Classic Forehead Lift

Before the operation begins, your hair will be tied with rubber bands on either side of the incision line. Your head will not be shaved, but hair that is growing directly in front of the incision line may need to be trimmed.

For most patients, a coronal incision will be used. It follows a headphone-like pattern, starting at about ear level and running across the top of the forehead and down the other side of the head. The incision is usually made well behind the hairline so that the scar won't be visible.

If your hairline is high or receding, the incision may be placed just at the hairline, to avoid adding even more height to the forehead. In patients who are bald or losing hair, a mid-scalp incision that follows the natural pattern of the skull bones is sometimes recommended. By wearing your hair down on your forehead, most such scars become relatively inconspicuous. Special planning is sometimes necessary for concealing the scar in male patients, whose hairstyles often don't lend themselves as well to incision coverage.

If you are bald or have thinning hair, your surgeon may recommend a mid-scalp incision so the resulting scar follows the natural junction of two bones in your skull and is less conspicuous.

Working through the incision, the skin of the forehead is carefully lifted so that the underlying tissue can be removed and the muscles of the forehead can be altered or released. The eyebrows may also be elevated and excess skin at the incision point will be trimmed away to help create a smoother, more youthful appearance.

Your face and hair will be washed to prevent irritation and the rubber bands will be removed from your hair. Although some plastic surgeons do not use any dressings, your doctor may choose to cover the incision with gauze padding and wrap the head in an elastic bandage.

The Endoscopic Forehead Lift

Typically, an endoscopic forehead lift requires the same preparation steps as the traditional procedure: the hair is tied back and trimmed behind the hairline where the incisions will be made.

However, rather than making one long coronal incision, your surgeon will make three, four or five short scalp incisions, each less than an inch in length. An endoscope, which is a pencil-like camera device connected to a television monitor, is inserted through one of the incisions, allowing the surgeon to have a clear view of the muscles and tissues beneath the skin. Using another instrument inserted through a different incision, the forehead skin is lifted and the muscles and underlying tissues are removed or altered to produce a smoother appearance. The eyebrows may also be lifted and secured into their higher position by sutures beneath the skin's surface or by temporary fixation screws placed behind the hairline.

When the lift is complete, the scalp incisions will be closed with stitches or clips and the area will be washed. Gauze and an elastic bandage may also be used, depending on your surgeon's preference.

After Your Surgery

The immediate post-operative experience for a patient who has had a classic forehead lift may differ significantly from a patient who had the procedure performed endoscopically.

Classic forehead lift patients may experience some numbness and temporary discomfort around the incision, which can be controlled with prescription medication. Patients who are prone to headaches may be treated with an additional longer-acting local anesthesia during surgery as a preventive measure.

You may be told to keep your head elevated for two to three days following surgery to keep the swelling down. Swelling may also affect the cheeks and eyes—however, this should begin to disappear in a week or so.

As the nerves heal, numbness on the top of your scalp may be replaced by itching. These sensations may take as long as six months to fully disappear. If bandages were used, they will be removed a day or two after surgery. Most stitches or clips will be removed within two weeks, sometimes in two stages.

Some of your hair around the incision may fall out and may temporarily be a bit thinner. Normal growth will usually resume within a few weeks or months. Permanent hair loss is rare.

Endoscopic forehead lift patients may experience some numbness, incision discomfort and mild swelling.

Incision site pain is usually minimal, but can be controlled with medication, if necessary. Endoscopic forehead lift patients usually experience less of the itching sensation felt by patients who have had the classic forehead lift. The stitches or staples used to close the incisions are usually removed within a week and the temporary fixation screws within two weeks.

Getting Back to Normal

Although you should be up and about in a day or two, plan on taking it easy for at least the first week after surgery. You should be able to shower and shampoo your hair within two days, or as soon as the bandage is removed.

Most patients are back to work or school in a week to 10 days. Endoscopic patients may feel ready to return even sooner. Vigorous physical activity should be limited for several weeks, including jogging, bending, heavy housework, sex, or any activity that increases your blood pressure. Prolonged exposure to heat or sun should be limited for several months.

Most of the visible signs of surgery should fade completely within about three weeks. Minor swelling and bruising can be concealed with special camouflage makeup. You may feel a bit tired and let down at first, but your energy level will increase as you begin to look and feel better.

Your New Look

Most patients are pleased with the results of a forehead lift, no matter which surgical method was used. Often, patients don't realize how much their sagging forehead contributed to the signs of aging until they see how much younger and more rested they appear after the lift.

Although a forehead lift does not stop the clock, it can minimize the appearance of aging for years. As time passes, you may want to repeat the procedure.

FAQs are available on Face Lift Surgery and Blepharoplasty (Eyelid Surgery). Procedural information is also available for Facelift and Eyelid Surgery.

Additional information on plastic surgery is available from the Plastic Surgery Information Service web site at www.plasticsurgery.org or call (800) 635-0635.

Chapter 20

Laser Resurfacing

What Is Skin Resurfacing?

For years, dermatologic surgeons have searched for an ideal method for eliminating wrinkles, correcting acne scars and improving aging and sun-damaged skin. Laser resurfacing of the face is the latest scientific breakthrough in skin rejuvenation.

Using a wand-like laser handpiece, undesired skin cells and wrinkles literally disappear in a puff of mist and are replaced by fresh skin cells. Sometimes called "laser peeling," one of its most significant advantages over traditional techniques for skin resurfacing is that treatment is relatively bloodless. The procedure also offers more control in the depth of penetration of the skin's surface, and allows a new degree of precision and safety in treating delicate areas, such as on or near the lips and around the eyes.

Who Is Qualified to Perform Laser Resurfacing

Traditionally the experts in skin care and skin diseases, dermatologic surgeons have extensive experience with laser surgery and were among the first specialists to pioneer the use of lasers for treating a variety of skin disorders. In fact, the latest advances in laser resurfacing technology were pioneered and refined by dermatologic surgeons. Since results are technique-sensitive and entail an artistic

American Society for Dermatologic Surgery, Form No. #007 1996. © 1995-1999; reprinted with permission.

component, it's important to select a dermatologic surgeon with demonstrated laser expertise.

What Conditions Can Laser Resurfacing Treat?

Laser resurfacing is performed in the dermatologic surgeon's office to help:

- Erase fine lines and wrinkles of the face, especially on the upper lip, cheeks and forehead,
- Smooth and tighten eyelid skin,
- Improve crow's feet around the eyes,
- Soften pucker marks and frown lines,
- Remove brown spots and splotchy, uneven skin color,
- Improve and flatten scars, and
- Repair smoker's lines.

What Are the Benefits of Laser Surgery For Facial Resurfacing?

Laser resurfacing may offer you and your dermatologic surgeon the following general benefits:

- Improved treatment results,
- Relatively "bloodless" surgery,
- Precisely controlled surgery,
- An addition or alternative to other skin rejuvenating procedures, and
- Safe, reliable and effective out-patient, same-day surgery.

What Can be Expected During and After Laser Resurfacing?

Depending on the specific condition being treated, patients may receive a topical anesthetic cream with mild sedation, or local anesthesia, or monitored intravenous sedation. Discomfort is usually minor both during the procedure and throughout the recovery phase.

The time required to complete the procedure is generally between one and two hours, although this may vary depending on the sites treated.

Following skin resurfacing, the treated areas usually are kept moist with ointment or occlusive dressings (surgical bandages) for the first few days. The skin is typically red or pink and may be covered with a fine crust. The treated sites must be protected from sunlight after the procedure. Once healing is completed, sunblock lotion should be applied. Depending on the type of laser used and the individual's ability to heal, a pink surface color may remain for several days to several months. Makeup can be worn after about 7 to 14 days.

What Are the Possible Complications of the Procedure?

All surgical procedures carry some degree of risk. With the new Er:YAG and CO_2 laser surgery, the risk of scarring is low. Common side-effects may include crusting, mild swelling, redness or brown discoloration at the treatment sites. Some patients may require bleaching creams to help regulate skin color following laser resurfacing. Significant pain, bleeding, swelling and infection seldom occur and can be minimized by surgical techniques and vigorous postoperative care. These surgical techniques and pre-and post-operative regimes have been pioneered by dermatologic surgeons and continue to be enhanced and improved for patient safety and comfort.

What Are the Limitations of Laser Resurfacing?

Laser resurfacing is not a substitute for a facelift, nor can the procedure eliminate excessive skin or jowls. However, beneficial tightening of loose skin can occur from laser resurfacing, resulting in an improvement of certain folds and creases. In many cases, laser resurfacing offers an alternative to traditional methods for skin rejuvenation, such as dermabrasion and deep chemical peels. It can also work well in conjunction with or as an additional treatment to other aesthetic procedures, such as chemical peels, blepharoplasty (eyelid surgery) and liposuction of the face and neck.

For More Information

For more information on laser treatments and to obtain a referral list of laser experts in your geographic area, call the American Society for Dermatologic Surgery's toll-free consumer hotline, 1-800-441-2737, during weekday business hours (CST) or visit our Web site at www.asds-net.org.

The American Society for Dermatologic Surgery (ASDS)

The ASDS provides grants, training and continuing education for its members in new dermatologic surgical techniques and procedures. Represented in the American Medical Association House of Delegates, the Society was formed in 1970 to promote excellence in the subspecialty of dermatologic surgery and to foster the highest standards of patient care.

Chapter 21

Chemical Peeling

What Is Chemical Peeling?

Chemical peeling is a technique used to improve the appearance of the skin. In this treatment, a chemical solution is applied to the skin which causes it to separate and eventually peel off. The new, regenerated skin is usually smoother and less wrinkled than the old skin. The new skin is also more even in color.

Thousands of chemical peels are performed each year. Dermatologic surgeons have used various peeling agents for the last 100 years and are experts in performing multiple types of chemical peels. Today, with the public's increasing interest in rejuvenating skin and slowing the effects of the aging process, chemical peeling has emerged as an exciting supplement to a total skin care program. A thorough evaluation by your dermatologic surgeon is imperative before embarking upon a chemical peel.

What Can a Chemical Peel Do?

Chemical peeling is often used to treat fine lines under the eyes and around the mouth. Wrinkles caused by sun damage, aging and hereditary factors can often be reduced or even eliminated with this procedure. However, sags, bulges and more severe wrinkles do not respond well to peeling and may require other kinds of cosmetic

American Society for Dermatologic Surgery, Form No. 003 1994. © 1995-1999; reprinted with permission.

surgical procedures, such as an eyelid lift or soft tissue filler. A dermatologic surgeon can help determine the most appropriate type of treatment for each individual case.

Mild scarring and certain types of acne can be treated with chemical peels. In addition, pigmentation of the skin in the form of sun spots, age spots, liver spots, freckles, blotchiness due to taking birth control pills, and skin that is dull in texture and color may be improved with chemical peeling. Areas of sun-damaged skin, spots of precancerous keratoses and scaling patches may improve after chemical peeling. Following treatment, new lesions or patches are less likely to appear.

How Are Chemical Peels Performed?

The procedure can be performed on the face, neck, chest, hands, arms, and legs. Superficial, medium, or deep chemical peels may be used to improve damaged skin. As a rule, the deeper the peel, the longer the recovery time. Your dermatologic surgeon will recommend the best peel for your skin problems.

Prior to treatment, instructions may include stopping certain medications and preparing the skin with pre-conditioning creams.

A chemical peel can be performed in a dermatologic surgeon's office or in a surgery center as an out-patient procedure. The skin is thoroughly cleansed with an agent that removes excess oils, and the eyes and hair are protected. One or more chemical solutions—such as glycolic acid, trichloroacetic acid, salicylic acid, lactic acid, or carbolic acid (phenol)—are used. Your dermatologic surgeon will select the proper peeling agent based upon the type of skin damage present.

During a chemical peel, the physician applies the solution to various areas of the skin. These applications produce separation and eventual peeling of layers of skin, enabling new, regenerated skin to appear.

During the procedure, most patients experience a warm to somewhat hot sensation which lasts about 5 to 10 minutes, followed by a stinging sensation. A deeper peel may require pain medication during or after the procedure.

After Treatment, What Should Be Expected?

Depending upon the type of peel, a reaction similar to a mild to severe sunburn occurs following a chemical peel. Superficial peeling usually involves redness, followed by scaling that ends within three to five days.

Medium-depth and deep peeling can sometimes result in swelling and blisters that may break, crust, turn brown, and peel off over a period of 7 to 14 days. Some peels may require surgical tape to be placed on part or all of the skin that is treated.

It is important to avoid overexposure to the sun immediately after a chemical peel since the new skin is fragile and more susceptible to injury. Your dermatologic surgeon will prescribe proper follow-up care to help the skin through the healing stages.

What Are the Possible Complications?

In certain skin types, there is a risk of developing a temporary or permanent color change in the skin. Taking birth control pills, pregnancy, or a family history of brownish discoloration on the face may increase the possibility of developing abnormal pigmentation.

Although low, there is a risk of scarring after chemical peels. If scarring does occur, it can usually be treated with good results.

There is a small incidence of the reactivation of cold sores or herpes simplex infection in patients with a history of fever blisters.

Prior to a chemical peel, it is important for a patient to inform the physician of any past history of keloids, unusual scarring tendencies, extensive x-rays or radiation to the face, or recurring cold sores.

What Are the Limitations of Chemical Peels?

Chemical peels cannot remove loose or sagging skin and do not serve the same function as a face lift, brow lift, or eyelid lift. They do not eliminate the gravitational forces that produce loose skin.

Chemical peeling will not remove deep scars. Dermabrasion, punch grafting, punch elevation, scar excision, or soft tissue fillers may be much more effective for scars and should be discussed with your dermatologic surgeon.

Chemical peels cannot change pore size, nor can they predictably remove broken blood vessels on the face. However, chemical peels may improve the appearance of these conditions.

For More Information

For more information on skin conditions and chemical peels, consult your physician or call the American Society for Dermatologic Surgery's toll-free hotline, 1-800-441-2737, during weekday business hours (CST) or visit our Web site at www.asds-net.org . A referral list of dermatologic surgeons in your geographic area, along with chemical peel information, will be mailed upon request.

The American Society for Dermatologic Surgery (ASDS)

The ASDS provides research grants, training and continuing education for its members in new dermatologic surgical techniques and procedures. Represented in the American Medical Association House of Delegates, the ASDS was formed in 1970 to promote the highest standards of patient care for the surgical treatment of the skin, hair, nails, veins, and mucous membranes.

Chapter 22

Dermabrasion and Dermaplaning— Refinishing the Skin

If You're Considering a Skin-Refinishing Treatment

Dermabrasion and dermaplaning help to "refinish" the skin's top layers through a method of controlled surgical scraping. The treatments soften the sharp edges of surface irregularities, giving the skin a smoother appearance.

Dermabrasion is most often used to improve the look of facial skin left scarred by accidents or previous surgery, or to smooth out fine facial wrinkles, such as those around the mouth. It's also sometimes used to remove the pre-cancerous growths called keratoses. Dermaplaning is commonly used to treat deep acne scars.

Both dermabrasion and dermaplaning can be performed on small areas of skin or on the entire face. They can be used alone, or in conjunction with other procedures such as facelift, scar removal or revision, or chemical peel.

If you're considering surgery to refinish the skin, this text will give you a basic understanding of the procedure—when it can help, how it's performed, and what results you can expect. It can't answer all of your questions, since a lot depends on your individual circumstances. Please ask your doctor about anything you don't understand.

Considering Alternative Procedures

If you're planning "surface repairs" on your face, you may also be

American Society of Plastic Surgeons, reprinted from The Plastic Surgery Information Service at www.plasticsurgery.org. © 1994; reprinted with permission.

115

considering chemical peel, an alternative method of surgically removing the top layer of skin. However, dermabrasion and dermaplaning use surgical instruments to remove the affected skin layers, while chemical peel uses a caustic solution.

Many plastic surgeons perform all three procedures, selecting one or a combination of procedures to suit the individual patient and the problem. Others prefer one technique for all surface repairs. In general, chemical peel is used more often to treat fine wrinkles, and dermabrasion and dermaplaning for deeper imperfections such as acne scars. A non-chemical approach may also be preferred for individuals with slightly darker skin, especially when treating limited areas of the face, since dermabrasion and dermaplaning are less likely to produce extreme changes and contrasts in skin color. If you'd like more information on chemical peel, ask your plastic surgeon for the American Society of Plastic Surgeons (ASPS) brochure on that topic.

The Best Candidates for Dermabrasion

Dermabrasion and dermaplaning can enhance your appearance and your self-confidence, but neither treatment will remove all scars and flaws or prevent aging. Before you decide to have a skin-refinishing treatment, think carefully about your expectations and discuss them with your surgeon.

Men and women of all ages, from young people to older adults, can benefit from dermabrasion and dermaplaning. Although older people heal more slowly, more important factors are your skin type, coloring, and medical history. For example, black skin, Asian skin, and other dark complexions may become permanently discolored or blotchy after a skin-refinishing treatment. People who develop allergic rashes or other skin reactions, or who get frequent fever blisters or cold sores, may experience a flare-up. If you have freckles, they may disappear in the treated area.

In addition, most surgeons won't perform treatment during the active stages of acne because of a greater risk of infection. The same may be true if you've had radiation treatments, a bad skin burn, or a previous chemical peel.

All Surgery Carries Some Uncertainty and Risk

Dermabrasion and dermaplaning are normally safe when they're performed by a qualified, experienced board-certified physician. The most common risk is a change in skin pigmentation. Permanent darkening of the skin, usually caused by exposure to the sun in the days or months following surgery, may occur in some patients. On the other hand, some patients find the treated skin remains a little lighter or blotchy in appearance.

You may develop tiny whiteheads after surgery. These usually disappear on their own, or with the use of an abrasive pad or soap; occasionally, the surgeon may have to remove them. You may also develop enlarged skin pores; these usually shrink to near normal size once the swelling has subsided.

While infection and scarring are rare with skin-refinishing treatments, they are possible. Some individuals develop excessive scar tissue (keloid or hypertrophic scars); these are usually treated with the application or injection of steroid medications to soften the scar. You can reduce your risks by choosing a qualified plastic surgeon and closely following his or her advice.

Planning Your Surgery

Because these treatments have sometimes been offered by inadequately trained practitioners, it's especially important that you find a doctor (generally a plastic surgeon or a dermatologist) who is trained and experienced in the procedure. After all, dermabrasion and dermaplaning usually involve the most visible part of your body—your face.

In your initial consultation, be open in discussing your expectations with your surgeon, and don't hesitate to ask any questions or express any concerns you may have. Your surgeon should be equally open with you, explaining the factors that could influence the procedure and the results—such as your age, skin condition, and previous plastic surgeries.

The surgeon will discuss your medical history, conduct a routine examination, and photograph your face. He or she should explain the procedure in detail, along with its risks and benefits, the recovery period, and the costs. Insurance usually doesn't cover cosmetic procedures, however, it may cover dermabrasion or dermaplaning when performed to remove precancerous skin growths or extensive scars. Check your policy or call your carrier to be sure.

Preparing for Your Surgery

Your surgeon will give you specific instructions on how to prepare for surgery, including guidelines on eating and drinking, and on avoiding aspirin and other medications that affect blood clotting. You may also be given special instructions regarding the care and treatment of your skin prior to surgery. If you smoke, you'll probably be asked to stop for a week or two before and after surgery, since smoking decreases blood circulation in the skin and impedes healing. While you're making preparations, be sure to arrange for someone to drive you home after your surgery, and to help you out for a day or two if needed.

Where Your Surgery will be Performed

Your treatment may be performed in a surgeon's office-based facility, an outpatient surgery center, or a hospital. It's usually done on an outpatient basis, for cost containment and convenience. However, if you're undergoing extensive work, you may be admitted to the hospital.

Types of Anesthesia

Dermabrasion and dermaplaning may be performed under local anesthesia, which numbs the area, combined with a sedative to make you drowsy. You'll be awake but relaxed, and will feel minimal discomfort. Sometimes a numbing spray, such as freon, is used along with or instead of local anesthesia. Or, in more severe cases, your surgeon may prefer to use general anesthesia, in which case you'll sleep through the procedure.

The Surgery

Dermabrasion and dermaplaning can be performed fairly quickly. The procedures usually take from a few minutes to an hour and a half, depending on how large an area of skin is involved. It's not uncommon for the procedure to be performed more than once, or in stages, especially when scarring is deep or a large area of skin is involved.

In dermabrasion, the surgeon scrapes away the outermost layer of skin with a rough wire brush, or a burr containing diamond particles, attached to a motorized handle. The scraping continues until the surgeon reaches the safest level that will make the scar or wrinkle less visible.

In dermaplaning, the surgeon uses a hand-held instrument called a dermatome. Resembling an electric razor, the dermatome has an oscillating blade that moves back and forth to evenly "skim" off the surface layers of skin that surround the craters or other facial defects. This skimming continues until the lowest point of the acne scar becomes more even with the surrounding skin.

The surgeon may then treat the skin in a number of ways, including ointment, a wet or waxy dressing, dry treatment, or some combination of these.

After Your Surgery

Right after the procedure, your skin will be quite red and swollen, and eating and talking may be difficult. You'll probably feel some tingling, burning, or aching; any pain you feel can be controlled with medications prescribed by your surgeon. The swelling will begin to subside in a few days to a week.

If you remember the scrapes you got when you fell down as a child, you'll have an idea of what to expect from this type of surgery. A scab or crust will form over the treated area as it begins to heal. This will fall off as a new layer of tight, pink skin forms underneath. Your face may itch as new skin starts to grow, and your surgeon may recommend an ointment to make you more comfortable. If ointment is applied immediately after surgery, little or no scab will form.

In any case, your surgeon will give you detailed instructions to care for your skin after surgery. For men, this will include delaying shaving for a while, then using an electric razor at first. It's very important that you understand your doctor's instructions and follow them exactly, to ensure the best possible healing.

If you notice the treated area beginning to get worse instead of better—for example, if it becomes increasingly red, raised, and itchy after it has started to heal—it may be a sign that abnormal scars are beginning to form. Call your surgeon as soon as possible, so that treatment can begin early.

Getting Back to Normal

Your new skin will be a bit swollen, sensitive, and bright pink for several weeks. During this time, you can begin gradually resuming your normal activities.

You can expect to be back at work in about two weeks. Your surgeon will probably advise your to avoid any activity that could cause a bump to your face for at least two weeks. More active sports—especially ball sports—should be avoided for four to six weeks. If you swim, stick to indoor pools to avoid sun and wind, and keep your face out of chlorinated water for at least four weeks. It will be at least three to four weeks before you can drink alcohol without experiencing a flush of redness.

Above all, it's important to protect your skin from the sun until the pigment has completely returned to your skin, as long as six to 12 months.

Your New Look

Refinishing treatments can offer dramatic improvements in the surface of your skin, but it will take some time before you see the final results. The pinkness of your skin will take about three months to fade. In the meantime, you'll probably want to wear non-allergenic makeup when you go out. (For tips on hiding your condition while it heals, ask your surgeon for the ASPS brochure on camouflage cosmetics.) When your new skin is fully re-pigmented, the color should closely match the surrounding skin, making the procedure virtually undetectable.

Additional information on plastic surgery is available from the Plastic Surgery Information Service web site at www.plasticsurgery.org or call (800) 635-0635.

Chapter 23

Understanding Blepharoplasty: Surgery of the Eyelids

Every year, 100,000 men and women choose blepharoplasty to improve the way they look. Droopy eyelids can make you look older and can also impair vision. Blepharoplasty corrects these problems and also removes puffiness and bags under the eyes that make you look worn and tired. This procedure cannot alter dark circles, fine lines and wrinkles around the eyes, nor can it change sagging eyebrows. Though blepharoplasty is often performed as a single procedure, your surgeon may also recommend a browlift, facelift, or skin resurfacing to achieve the best results.

If you are wondering how blepharoplasty can change the way you look, you need to know how eyelid surgery is performed and what you can expect from this procedure. This chapter can address many common questions and provide you the information to begin considering blepharoplasty.

Successful facial plastic surgery is a result of good rapport between patient and surgeon. Trust, based on realistic expectations and exacting medical expertise, develops in the consulting stages before surgery. Your surgeon can answer specific questions about your specific needs.

As with all facial plastic surgery, good health and realistic expectations are prerequisites. Blepharoplasty removes the excess fat,

American Academy of Facial Plastic and Reconstructive Surgery reprinted from http://www.facial-plastic-surgery.org. © 1996 American Academy of Facial Plastic and Reconstructive Surgery; reprinted with permission.

muscle and skin from both upper and lower lids. The results can be a refreshed appearance, with a younger, firmer eye area.

People with circulatory, ophthalmological, or serious medical conditions must rely on the diagnostic skills of their own personal specialists to determine whether blepharoplasty is an option to consider. Consultation with the facial plastic surgeon can help you decide whether any additional, complementary surgery would increase the success of the surgery. Your surgeon might recommend planning a simultaneous forehead lift to correct a drooping brow and smooth the forehead, or skin resurfacing to remove the fine line wrinkling in the eye area.

Making the Decision for Blepharoplasty

Whether the surgery is desired for functional or cosmetic reasons, your choice of a qualified facial plastic surgeon is of paramount importance. The patient must also make the commitment to follow the pre-surgical and post-operative instructions of the surgeon.

During the pre-surgical consultation, you will be examined or asked to answer queries concerning vision, tear production, use of lenses, and your desires for surgery. Your surgeon will explain what you can expect from blepharoplasty and take a complete medical history. Factors to be weighed include age, skin type, ethnic background, and degree of vision obstruction. Furthermore, you can expect an open and honest exchange between you and your surgeon, which will establish the basis for a successful outcome.

After a mutual decision is made by both you and your surgeon, the technique indicated for your individual surgery will be discussed. The type of anesthesia, the surgical facility, any supportive surgery, and the risks and costs inherent in the procedure will be outlined.

Understanding the Surgery

In upper eyelid surgery, the surgeon first marks the individual lines and creases of the lids in order to keep the scars as invisible as possible along these natural folds. The incision is made, and excess fat, muscle, and loose skin are removed. Fine sutures are used to close the incisions, thereby minimizing the visibility of any scar.

In lower eyelid surgery, the surgeon makes the incision in an inconspicuous site along the lashline and smile creases of the lower lid. Excess fat, muscle and skin are then trimmed away before the incision is closed with fine sutures. Eyelid puffiness caused primarily by excess fat may be corrected by a transconjunctival blepharoplasty. The incision in this case is made inside the lower eyelid, and excess fatty material is removed. When sutures are used to close this kind of incision, they are invisible to the eye. They are also self-dissolving and leave no visible scar. Under normal conditions, blepharoplasty can take from one to two hours.

What to Expect after the Surgery

Immediately after the surgery has been completed, your surgeon may apply tiny sterile bandages. This is not done for transconjunctival blepharoplasty. It is not crucial that the eyes be covered. However, an ointment to prevent dryness of the eye area may be used. A certain degree of swelling and bruising is normal. Cold compresses, as well as head elevation when lying down, will enhance healing and relieve discomfort. Your surgeon will prescribe medication for discomfort.

For a week and a half following blepharoplasty, you will clean the eye area (the eyes may feel sticky, dry, and itchy). Eyedrops may be recommended. Your surgeon will also list activities and environments to avoid in the weeks immediately following surgery. Permanent stitches will be removed in three to five days after surgery. Self-absorbing stitches will dissolve on their own.

Facial plastic surgery makes it possible to correct many facial flaws and signs of premature aging that can undermine self-confidence. By changing how you look, facial plastic surgery can help change how you feel about yourself.

Insurance does not generally cover surgery that is done purely for cosmetic reasons. Surgery to correct or improve vision or surgery for eye deformity or injury may be reimbursable in whole or in part. It is the patient's responsibility to check with the insurance carrier for information on the degree of coverage.

For more information write or call the AAFPRS at 310 S. Henry Street, Alexandria, Virginia 22314, (703) 299-9291, 1-800-332-FACE. Or visit their web site at from http://www.facial-plastic-surgery.org.

Chapter 24

Facial Implants

Facial implants are used to improve and enhance facial contours. They are used for example to reshape the chin or nose or improve the look of sunken cheekbones.

Most of the facial implant procedures are performed in an office-based facility, an outpatient surgical center or a hospital outpatient facility. They may be done alone or combined with other procedures on the face. Facial implant surgery is done under local or general anesthesia.

Chin implant surgery is used to augment a weak chin. The purpose is to bring it into balance with other facial features. This procedure is done as an outpatient procedure under local anesthesia. It may take from 30 minutes to an hour. The small incision to insert the implant is placed inside the mouth or in the skin just under the chin area. The scar resulting from this incision is usually not noticeable. Normal activity can be resumed within a week after this procedure.

Cheek implant surgery is used to produce a stronger profile and more pronounced cheeks It usually takes about 30 to 60 minutes. The implant is inserted through an incision made either inside the upper lip or the lower eyelid. If this procedure is performed in combination with another face procedure the implant is inserted through any of the other incisions. Normal activity can be resumed in two or three days.

Jaw implant surgery usually takes about one to two hours. Incisions are made on either side of the lower lip to insert the implant.

Lip augmentation is done by inserting lip implants to achieve voluptuous lips. This procedure is performed as an out-patient procedure. Local anesthesia is usually used. The procedure takes about an hour. Normal activity can be resumed in about one week.

Facial implant surgery is generally a safe procedure when performed by a qualified plastic surgeon. See "How to Choose a Plastic Surgeon" for additional information about getting qualified medical assistance. As with any surgical procedure, there are some risks which should be discussed with your surgeon.

For additional information and/or personal consultation, you can find the plastic surgeon nearest you in Plastic Surgeon Locator at http://www.plastic-surgery.net, provided by the Plastic Surgery Network.

Chapter 25

Hair Replacement Surgery

Hair replacement surgery is used to correct the hair loss in either men or women. Aging, change in hormones, and a family history of baldness are the most common causes of hair loss. Certain medications, burns and trauma can also result in hair loss.

All hair replacement techniques are based on finding the most efficient use of your existing hair. Grafts or flaps are taken from the healthy hair growth at the back and sides of the head.

There are several techniques for hair replacement. Hair transplant techniques using grafts are the most common and can take a long time to complete, up to two years. Flaps, tissue-expansion and scalp-reduction procedures are more extensive procedures but they produce dramatic change in a shorter time.

In hair transplantation small pieces of hair-bearing scalp grafts are taken from a donor site and relocated into a bald or thinning area. There are different kinds of grafts depending on their size and shape. Punch grafts (about 10-15 hairs.); mini-graft (about two to four hairs); the micro-graft (one to two hairs.); slit grafts (four to 10 hairs); and strip grafts (30-40 hairs.) The smaller the number of hairs in the graft the more natural look it will produce.

In tissue expansion technique, a balloon-like device is inserted beneath hair-bearing scalp and the device is gradually inflated with salt water over a period of weeks. This allows the gradual expansion

"Hair Replacement Surgery" reprinted from Plastic Surgery Network at http://www.plastic-surgery.net. © 1997-2000 Medical-Web Network; reprinted with permission.

of the skin and the growth of new skin cells. The expanded skin is used in another procedure to cover the bald area.

Flap surgery: This procedure is used to quickly cover large areas of baldness. After cutting out a section of the bald scalp, a flap of the hair-bearing part of the scalp is lifted of the surface while still attached at one end and brought into the new position and sewn into place. The attached end of the flap supplies the blood supply to the new area.

Scalp reduction: This technique is used to cover the bald areas at the top and back of the head. In this procedure a segment of bald scalp is removed under local anesthesia. The hair bearing skin surrounding the cut-out area is then loosened and pulled together to close the defect.

Combining scalp reduction with tissue expansion and flap surgery can sometimes be used to achieve the best results.

Although hair replacement surgery is normally safe, as with any surgical procedure, there are some risks which should be discussed with your surgeon.

Hair replacement surgery is usually performed as an outpatient procedure in a physician's office, in an outpatient surgery center, or a hospital. It is usually performed using local anesthesia. Cases involving tissue expansion, scalp reduction or flaps may need general anesthesia.

For additional information and /or personal consultation, you can find the plastic surgeon nearest you in Plastic Surgeon Locator at http://www.plastic-surgery.net, provided by the Plastic Surgery Network.

Chapter 26

Understanding Rhinoplasty: Surgery of the Nose

Every year, 500,000 people who are interested in improving the appearance of their noses seek consultation with facial plastic surgeons. Some are unhappy with the noses they were born with, and some with the way aging has changed their nose. For others, an injury may have distorted the nose, or the goal may be improved breathing. But one thing is clear: nothing has a greater impact on how a person looks than the size and shape of the nose. Because the nose is the most defining characteristic of the face, a slight alteration can greatly improve one's appearance.

If you have wondered how nose surgery, or rhinoplasty, could improve your looks, self-confidence, or health, you need to know how rhinoplasty is performed and what you can expect. No article can answer all your concerns, but this one can provide answers to many of the questions you may have.

Successful facial plastic surgery is a result of good rapport between patient and surgeon. Trust, based on realistic expectations and exacting medical expertise, develops in the consulting stages before surgery. Your surgeon can answer specific questions about your specific needs.

Is Rhinoplasty for You?

As with all facial plastic surgery, good health and realistic expectations are prerequisites. Understanding nose surgery is also critical.

American Academy of Facial Plastic and Reconstructive Surgery reprinted from http://www.facial-plastic-surgery.org. © 1996, American Academy of Facial Plastic and Reconstructive Surgery; reprinted with permission.

Since there is no ideal in rhinoplasty, the goal is to improve the nose aesthetically, making it harmonize better with other facial features.

Skin type, ethnic background, and age are important factors to be considered in discussions with your surgeon prior to surgery. Before the nose is altered, a young patient must reach full growth, usually around age 15 or 16. Exceptions are cases in which breathing is severely impaired.

Before deciding on rhinoplasty, ask your facial plastic surgeon if any additional surgery might be recommended to enhance the appearance of your face. Many patients have chin augmentation in conjunction with rhinoplasty to create a better balance of features.

Making the Decision for Rhinoplasty

Whether the surgery is desired for functional or cosmetic reasons, your choice of a qualified facial plastic surgeon is of paramount importance. Many facial plastic surgeons are trained in both ear, nose, throat, and facial cosmetic surgery, which provides you, the patient, with the highest level of training and expertise. Your surgeon will examine the structure of your nose, both externally and internally, to evaluate what you can expect from rhinoplasty. Your surgeon will also discuss factors that may influence the outcome of the surgery, such as skin type, ethnic background, age, degree of deformity, and degree of function of nasal structures.

You can expect a thorough explanation of the surgeon's expectations and the risks involved in surgery. Following a joint decision by you and your surgeon to proceed with rhinoplasty, the surgeon will take photographs of you and discuss the options available. Your surgeon will explain how the nasal structures, including bone and cartilage, can be sculpted to reshape the nose and indicate how reshaping the chin, for example, could enhance the desired results.

After conducting a thorough medical history, your surgeon will offer information regarding anesthesia, the surgical facility to be used, and the costs for the procedure.

Understanding the Surgery

The definition of rhinoplasty is, literally, shaping the nose. First, incisions are made and the skin of the nose is lifted from its underlying bone and cartilage support system. The majority of incisions are made inside the nose, where they are invisible. In some cases, an incision is made in the area of skin separating the nostrils. Next, certain amounts of underlying bone and cartilage are removed or rearranged to provide a newly shaped structure. For example, when the tip of the nose is too large, the surgeon can sculpt the cartilage in this area to reduce it in size. The angle of the nose in relation to the upper lip can be altered for a more youthful look or to correct a distortion.

The skin is then redraped over the new frame and the incisions are closed. A splint is applied to the outside of the nose to help retain the new shape while the nose heals. Soft, absorbent material may be used inside the nose to maintain stability along the dividing wall of the air passages called the septum. Risk factors in rhinoplasty are generally minor, and your facial plastic surgeon will discuss these prior to surgery.

What to Expect

Immediately after surgery, a small splint will be placed on your nose to protect it and to keep the structure stable for at least five to eight days. If packing is placed inside the nose during surgery, it is removed the morning following the surgery. Your face will feel puffy, especially the first day after surgery. Pain medication may be required. Your surgeon will advise you to avoid blowing your nose for seven days after surgery. In the immediate days following surgery, you may experience bruising and minor swelling in the eye area. Cold compresses often reduce the bruising and discomfort. Absorbable sutures are usually used that do not have to be removed. Nasal dressing and splints are usually removed six or seven days after surgery.

It is crucial that you follow your surgeon's directions, especially instructions to keep your head elevated for a certain period after surgery. Some activities will be prohibited in the weeks after the procedure. Sun exposure, exertion, and risk of injury must be avoided. If you wear glasses, special arrangements must be made to ensure that the glasses do not rest on the bridge of the nose. Tape and other devices are sometimes used to permit wearing glasses without stressing the area where surgery was performed.

Follow-up care is vital for this procedure to monitor healing. Obviously, anything unusual should be reported to your surgeon immediately. It is essential that you keep your follow-up appointments with your surgeon.

Insurance does not generally cover surgery that is purely for cosmetic reasons. Surgery to correct or improve nasal function or surgery for major deformity or injury may be reimbursable in whole or in part. It is the patient's responsibility to check with the insurance carrier for information on the degree of coverage.

For more information write or call the AAFPRS at 310 S. Henry Street, Alexandria, Virginia 22314, (703) 299-9291, 1-800-332-FACE. Or visit their web site at from http://www.facial-plastic-surgery.org.

Chapter 27

Ear Shaping (Otoplasty)

Otoplasty is an operation which is done to improve the appearance of the ears. It is most commonly done for protruding ears, often called "lop" ears or "cup" ears. The condition is often quite troubling to children who often take a great deal of kidding from their peers. Prior to the days when long hair was stylish, otoplasty was a very common operation. Parents seemed quite attuned to the problems faced by children with this condition. When long hair became stylish, the operation lost popularity, and has never seemed to become as popular as in the past. Perhaps with greater awareness, more parents will realize how important this correction can be to their children.

The operation is usually done during childhood, and this is ideal since the cartilage is still quite soft and malleable. We generally recommend that the procedure be done shortly before the child enters school. Adults also request this type of surgery having been denied the opportunity to have the deformity corrected during childhood. In these cases, the technique may be modified slightly to allow for softening of the cartilage in addition to reshaping.

The otoplasty operation consists of reshaping the cartilage of the ear, occasionally removing some cartilage, and placement of the ears in proper relationship to the face and head. It produces generally good cosmetic results. Even when results are occasionally imperfect, it is

Howard A. Tobin, M.D., F.A.C.S., Facial Plastic & Cosmetic Surgical Center, reprinted from the website at www.newlook.com. © 2000; reprinted with permission.

133

usually possible to make revisions successfully. The operation is carried out under either local or general anesthesia depending on the age and preference of the patient. There is relatively little pain associated with otoplasty and recovery is rapid. The incisions are made behind the ear where they are not noticeable. Absorbable sutures are used, making suture removal unnecessary.

A wraparound bandage is worn for a few days to protect the ears, and is worn at night until healing is complete. Most adult patients can return to work within a few days of surgery and children can return to school within a week. Trauma to the ears must be avoided for several weeks until healing is complete, and so a protective wrap is advisable during vigorous activity for at least three weeks.

Complications are uncommon. The major risk is postoperative bleeding. If this occurs, prompt treatment is required to prevent infection or abnormal scarring which can lead to thickening of the ear. Absolute symmetry of the ears is a goal that is rarely achieved. However, it is natural for the two ears to be slightly different in shape or position. Occasionally, after healing, the position of the ear can change, although the results of surgery are usually permanent.

For additional information contact: Howard A. Tobin, M.D., F.A.C.S., Facial Plastic & Cosmetic Surgical Center, 6300 Regional Plaza, Abilene, Texas 79606. (915) 695-3630; Toll Free (800) 592-4533; Fax (915) 695-3633; e-mail: n41gt@newlook.com.

Chapter 28

Breast Enlargement (Augmentation Mammoplasty)

It is estimated that more than 1.5 million women in this country have had augmentation mammoplasty. The procedure may be performed in several ways using intravenous sedation with local anesthesia or with general anesthesia. The incision may be placed in one of three locations: under the breast in the inframammary crease, under the areola (the colored skin around the nipple), or in the axilla (armpit).

Only the saline (saltwater) filled silicone breast implants can now be used for augmentation mammoplasty. The implants are available in a round or teardrop shape with a smooth or textured surface. The implant is placed under the breast tissue and on top of or under the pectoralis muscle. The final decision regarding which procedure to use will be made by you and your surgeon.

After the procedure, you will be advised regarding wound care, bra selection, suture removal and follow-up. You are asked to take it easy and remain quiet the night of surgery as bleeding around the implant can occasionally occur. It will take about three weeks for the swelling and discoloration to subside and to return to a normal lifestyle.

Postoperative bleeding is one complication. If this occurs, it will usually be within the first couple of days and may require another operation to remove the collection of blood (hematoma). Infection is very uncommon, but should it occur adjacent to the implant, it might be necessary to remove the implant to resolve the infection. In some breasts, firmness develops following surgery because of formation of scar tissue around the implant. This is called 'capsular contracture' and may require secondary surgery to correct. Sensation change around the nipple area can occur but in most cases is temporary. Difference between the shape of the breasts occasionally occurs.

In most cases, these problems can be treated with acceptable results. Since the implants are a plastic material, they can rupture and their contents leak. In the saline filled implants, rupture causes deflation. Rupture of the implant is very unusual and can be easily corrected with replacement of the implant. Occasionally, in scar tissue around the implant, calcium deposits can develop. These deposits may be seen on a mammography and can be distinguished from calcium deposits seen in breast cancer.

If corrective surgery is required within one year of the initial operation, there will be no surgeon's fee; however, the patient will be responsible for the operating room, anesthesia, and other miscellaneous charges. If the implant ruptures within one year of the initial operation, there will be no surgeon's fee for replacement of the implant. The patient is asked to cover the cost of the operating room, anesthesia, tests and implant. If the implant ruptures after one year the surgeon's fee will be reduced by 50 percent. Several implant manufacturers will replace the implant at no charge if there is a rupture.

After augmentation mammoplasty many patients have breastfed without difficulty. Occasionally, stretch marks develop.

Breast implants have never been shown to cause any form of cancer in women. Implants do make mammography somewhat less accurate and more difficult to interpret. If you are having a mammogram, advise your radiologist about your augmentation mammoplasty so the mammogram technique can be modified.

There have been extensive media reports and some medical reports of patients with implants developing a connective tissue or neurologic disease suggesting that there might be a connection between the two; however, we know of no scientific data to support this causal relationship. In addition, the media and some patients have raised the question of birth defects in children of mothers with breast implants. Because of these questions, the U.S. Food and Drug Administration has limited the use of silicone gel-filled implants for augmentation mammoplasty. Please obtain and read the manufacturer's information insert on any implant that you choose.

Recently, some health insurance providers are excluding coverage for breast disease if a patient has had breast implants. In spite of the potential problems, most women who have had this surgery are very happy with the results. They report feeling better about themselves and having more self-esteem.

There are several variations where incisions can be made: beneath the arm, under the breast, or around the nipple. The implant can be placed either on top of the pectoralis muscle or under the pectoralis muscle.

Chapter 29

Breast Lift (Mastopexy)

Breast sagging, or ptosis, as it is called medically, is a disturbing condition for women because it reflects the effects of aging and gravity on the breast position. The breasts appear droopy and less full than normal. The upper portion of the breasts appears flattened, and the lower portion descends below the crease beneath the breasts. Breast skin may often have reduced elasticity and become stretched or weakened.

Symmetrical and naturally proportioned and positioned breasts are the goals of breast elevation, or mastopexy, as the operation is technically named. A patients understanding and input will aid the surgeon in determining the proposed breast size, shape and position.

Indications

Many patients seek mastopexy following weight loss, pregnancy, lactation, or menopause. The presence of ptosis indicates the inelastic nature of the skin and a corresponding decrease in breast volume. In others, the normal aging process may result in a loss of breast tissue, which is of sufficient degree that correction is desired.

Because there are various degrees of ptosis, the surgical treatment involves a range of possible corrections based primarily on the nipple-areolar position, the amount of excess skin, and the breast volume.

Howard A. Tobin, M.D., F.A.C.S., Facial Plastic & Cosmetic Surgical Center, reprinted from the website at www.newlook.com. © 2000; reprinted with permission.

Correction may be as simple as breast augmentation. For minor degrees of ptosis, this adds fullness and may give added cleavage by increasing volume. The advantage of this approach is that it avoids visible scarring, since it is done through the tiny hidden incisions used in breast augmentation. Since breast augmentation only provides added fill, it does not truly lift the breast. It is important to understand this, since there is a common misconception that by filling the breast, there will automatically be lifting. Breast augmentation does nothing to correct the underlying condition of excess breast skin.

True mastopexy involves skin removal and, as a result, will require added incisions and scarring. The decision of the patient and the surgeon will always have to consider the willingness to accept these scars. While every effort is made to produce fine scars, this is often out of the control of the surgeon, and unsatisfactory scarring is a risk that cannot be avoided.

Types of Mastopexy

The simplest form of mastopexy involves removal of skin from around the areola (the dark skin around the nipple). This can also be used to decrease the size of the areola if it is already too large. The surrounding skin is then gathered and sutured to the areolar tissue. The scar is limited to around the areola, and since it is at the junction of the light and dark skin, it tends to be well camouflaged. This operation fell out of favor because invariably, there would be secondary stretching of the areola within a year of so of the operation. The technique has been modified to incorporate a purse string suture that supports the bunching up of tissue and has been very helpful in overcoming many of the problems of the original operation. Popularized by Dr. Louis Binelli, of Paris, this operation is now one of the most common types of mastopexy performed.

While it is attractive in its simplicity, there are distinct disadvantages. First of all, during the first year after surgery, there is a visible puckering and bunching around the incision. This is quite variable, but while it generally smoothes out, it is quite noticeable at first. More significantly, in the long term, the operation suffers from the fact that there remains a somewhat unnatural fullness beneath the breast and in the lateral quadrant that is the result of not removing skin from under the breast. Combining the lift with the use of a small implant minimizes some of these disadvantages. In our experience, this operation is usually carried out only in conjunction with augmentation. Not surprisingly, this is one of the most popular mastopexies, largely because of its relative simplicity and the avoidance of scars beneath the breast. As in all cases, it represents a compromise.

For more advanced ptosis, skin is removed from around the areola and from the bottom of the breast, allowing an upward repositioning of the nipple complex as well as a tightening of the lower breast. Although this leaves some scarring beneath the breast, the improvement in shape and firmness usually represents a satisfactory trade off. There are a variety of operations of this type, but a scar around the areola as well as a vertical scar running from the lower edge of the areola downward to the base of the breast characterize all of them. There is also an additional scar in the crease beneath the breast in many cases.

Even though mastopexy can provide significant improvement, there are definite limitations to the operation, and it is unrealistic to expect that the operation will give enough lift to produce ideal breast shape. Some droop is likely to persist in many cases regardless of the technique utilized.

In all cases, the proposed incisions will be reviewed prior to surgery. Often patients can decide on which technique they prefer, recognizing that the procedures with additional scars will usually provide better shape. Mastopexy is often combined with augmentation when additional fullness is required. After the elevation, a small implant is inserted to improve fullness. When considering this operation, patients should also have a good understanding of the risks of breast augmentation, covered elsewhere.

Complications

Breast elevation is a very gratifying procedure for the proper patient and is enjoyed by many women. Its limitations are primarily those of the scars that are inevitable in this type of surgery. Although every effort is made to produce fine scars, the incisions made beneath the breast have a tendency to widen or thicken in certain patients. Sometimes, incisions are slow to heal following this operation, although surprisingly, slow healing wounds may still result in very satisfactory scars. If they are not, later revision can be done under local anesthesia. It is usually best to wait about a year before considering revision, since the scars will improve with time.

Other possible complications include asymmetry of the breasts, infection, loss of sensitivity of the skin or nipple or skin necrosis. When breast augmentation is combined, there are the additional risks of this procedure. Furthermore, mastopexy must not be considered a treatment for breasts that are also too large. In these cases, breast reduction is required—a topic that is discussed separately.

The procedure generally takes one to two hours. The breasts are taped for several days with elastic tape to provide support. The recovery period is quite brief and the patient may return to light work a few days after surgery, although the final healing takes a while longer, depending on the extent of surgery and individual healing factors.

The desired shape will not be apparent for several weeks after surgery, and changes occur for several months. Furthermore, it is important to recognize that the cause of saggy breasts is poor skin elasticity. Therefore, as time goes on, the breasts may sag again. It is not uncommon for patients who have this operation to return years later for a second procedure.

For additional information contact: Howard A. Tobin, M.D., F.A.C.S., Facial Plastic & Cosmetic Surgical Center, 6300 Regional Plaza, Abilene, Texas 79606. (915) 695-3630; Toll Free (800) 592-4533; Fax (915) 695-3633; e-mail: n41gt@newlook.com

Chapter 30

Breast Reduction Often Good Medicine

"I'm amazed when I go shopping. I can buy a dress, not separates with the top four sizes larger. Most of all, the pain in my neck and back is gone." Breast size usually isn't considered an appropriate topic for social conversation. But for a woman suffering the medical and social consequences of having large, pendulous breasts, talking with someone who has undergone breast reduction can be a "life-changing experience," says Mary-Margaret Richardson, a public affairs specialist with the Food and Drug Administration (FDA) in St. Louis, Mo.

Before surgery, Richardson, 53, had adapted to a "lifetime of discomfort—bras that never fit and caused deep grooves in my shoulders, plus neck and back pain, heat rashes under my breasts in the summer, and ever-increasing stooping under the weight of them."

After talking with Kellie Feldman, a neighbor who had undergone breast reduction, Richardson decided to have the procedure done herself. "I had gone for a cancer screening several months earlier, and the doctor who did the examination looked at my rutted shoulders and asked whether I had ever thought of having reduction. The seed was planted then," Richardson said. "Then I talked with Kellie, and she was so positive about it."

Feldman, 27, is a special education teacher in St. Louis. "Actually, my father had been encouraging me to have the surgery," she says. "I was a bit put off, wondering why he was looking at my breasts. But

U.S. Food and Drug Administration, *FDA Consumer*, Jan-Feb 1997, Vol. 31, No. 1, pgs. 22(4).

he said that when I got older, they would look terrible. And I knew I already had deep shoulder indentations from my bra. In addition, the male students in school were always looking and commenting, which made me feel uncomfortable."

Margie, 40, an advertising executive in New York City who asked that her last name not be used, had a very different reason for undergoing breast reduction. "I have breast cancer and had a mastectomy on my right breast and then an implant," she says. "My surgeon recommended reduction for the left breast so that it would look more like the right."

Medical Concerns

Although very different from one another, these women share a mix of medical problems and cosmetic concerns that led them—and thousands of other women across the country—to undergo breast reduction surgery. "I can move my head and neck without pain, my shoulders have healed, and I just feel so much better," says Richardson. "I think about my grandmother, who had this problem all her life and was always stooped in pain. I wish she could have had something like this done then."

"Among my patients, I find there are certain age clusters with similar concerns," says George Beraka, M.D., a board-certified plastic and reconstructive surgeon who is assistant professor of surgery at Cornell Medical Center in New York City. "Those in their late teens realize they don't want to live with such large breasts. Women who have finished childbearing and breast-feeding say to themselves, 'Now I'd like to look and feel better.' And older women often are referred by their internists because of neck and back pain."

In some women, breast examination and mammography may be easier to perform after reduction. "From the standpoint of the physical exam, it may be more difficult to pick up a very small lesion [lump] in a woman with very large breasts," says Charles Finder, M.D., a radiologist in FDA's Mammography Quality and Radiation Program. "Imaging large breasts for mammography may be a bit more technically demanding, since the technician may have to get each view done twice, or do two images per view."

Richardson notes that she "kept getting abnormal mammograms with 'dense tissue' reports that made me think I had breast cancer." She is "looking forward to a normal result this time." But Finder cautions that this may not be the case. "If the breasts are reduced uniformly, then the tissue may still be dense, and she could still have problems with mammography," he says. Contraindications to the procedure "would apply to any major elective surgery," says Beraka. "The woman should not have any significant illness, either physical or mental."

Patricia McGuire, M.D., a board-certified plastic and reconstructive surgeon on staff at Parkcrest Surgical in St. Louis, says she prefers not to perform breast reduction on women who are heavy smokers because of a loss of blood supply, or on those with diabetes, since they may not heal well. Also, "if a woman is really overweight, I encourage her to get her weight down first. This is particularly a problem with teens with large breasts, since they may try to gain weight so that their bodies look more balanced," says McGuire, who performed the reductions for Richardson and Feldman.

Both physicians believe it is best to wait until a young woman's breasts are fully grown, usually by age 18, before doing a reduction. The procedure is not recommended for women who intend to breast-feed, according to the American Society of Plastic and Reconstructive Surgeons.

Breast Cancer

Concerns that breast reduction might increase the risk of breast cancer are unfounded, according to Beraka. "There are no data to suggest that women who undergo breast reduction are at greater risk for breast cancer, or that those with a family history of breast cancer should not have the procedure," says Beraka. "In fact, reduction is like a giant biopsy of the breast, because all tissue that is removed during surgery is examined by a pathologist."

During 20 years of performing the procedure, Beraka says, malignant tissue was found among his patients "maybe half a dozen times." McGuire, who has been performing reductions for five years, had one patient in whom cancerous tissue was discovered.

Preparing for Surgery

During the initial consultation, the surgeon explains the surgery in detail, including risks, limitations and scarring, which is an inevitable consequence of the procedure. The surgeon also discusses where the surgery will take place, how long the woman will remain in the facility, any steps that need to be taken preoperatively, and what to expect post-operatively. Any questions a woman has are answered at this time.

In preparation for surgery, the woman has a complete physical examination. The surgeon measures the woman's breasts and usually photographs them for reference during surgery and afterwards. These photographs can also serve as documentation for insurance purposes.

Unlike a rhinoplasty (nose reduction), in which computer imaging may be used to show a prospective patient what her nose is likely to look like after surgery, the new breast size and shape, as well as positioning of the nipple and areola (the darker skin around the nipple), are usually determined during a discussion between the physician and patient.

"Preoperative imaging of any sort is of limited value for this procedure. It's a marketing tool more than anything else," says Beraka. "After assessing the size of the breasts, I ask the patient how much smaller she would like them, taking into consideration what makes sense in terms of the rest of her body. I then estimate how much tissue will need to be removed."

Most surgeons provide guidelines for eating, drinking, smoking, taking medication, and other activities before surgery. Generally, the patient should not take aspirin or similar medications for a week or two before surgery, since these medications may lead to increased bleeding. Beraka suggests women take 1,000 milligrams of vitamin C daily to promote healing, but avoid vitamin E supplements, which may also lead to increased bleeding.

If a patient smokes, she may be advised to stop. This is always a good idea, but it's especially important when general anesthesia is used, since smoking limits the amount of oxygen the body has available during surgery and recovery.

Because the size, shape and amount of tissue in the breast will change after reduction, most women are advised to have a preoperative mammogram and a postoperative mammogram six months to a year after surgery for comparison.

The Surgery

Breast reduction is generally done on an inpatient basis. The procedure itself usually takes from two to four hours and requires an overnight stay in the hospital. In most cases, surgery is performed under general anesthesia. Generally, breast reduction involves the removal of fat, glandular tissue and skin from the breasts; in some cases, the areola may also be reduced.

Surgical techniques vary, but according to the American Society of Plastic and Reconstructive Surgeons, "the most common procedure involves an anchor shaped incision that circles the areola, extends downward, and follows the natural curve of the crease beneath the breast." After removing excess tissue and moving the nipple and areola into their new positions, the surgeon then "brings the skin from both sides of the breast down and around the areola, shaping the new contour of the breast."

Liposuction (a procedure in which excess fatty tissue is removed from a specific area of the body by means of a suction device) is sometimes used to remove excess fat from the armpit area, although some surgeons also use this procedure to remove excess fatty tissue from the breast. In some cases, if only fat needs to be removed, liposuction alone may be used to reduce breast size. The fatty tissue is also reviewed by a pathologist.

Beraka notes that newer surgical techniques, such as those popularized by Belgian surgeon Madeleine Lejour, can result in significantly less scarring around the undersurface of the breast, making the procedure "less frightening to patients contemplating reduction." However, McGuire says that while the Lejour technique can be appropriate "for specific patients," she does not believe it should be used for everyone. "The scars are shorter, but the surgeon has less control over the shape of the breast," she says. If the type of incision is important to the patient, she should discuss it with the surgeon.

Post-Op

After surgery, "they wrapped me in a bandage to hold everything in place," Richardson explains. "I was a bit uncomfortable, but I had very little pain. In fact, I never took anything stronger than extra-strength acetaminophen during recuperation."

The bandage is removed a couple of days after surgery, after which the woman wears a surgical bra 24 hours a day for about a month. "I could shower—I was up and active and doing things," says Richardson. Nevertheless, she took several weeks off from work to give her body a chance to recover before resuming a full schedule. Like most women who undergo reduction, Richardson was advised not to lift or push anything heavy for three or four weeks.

According to the American Society of Plastic and Reconstructive Surgeons, the first menstruation following surgery may cause breasts to swell and hurt, and the woman may also experience shooting pains in her breasts for several months. Patients may be advised to avoid sex for a week or so to avoid arousal that can cause the incisions to swell.

"I was relieved that my surgeon has an assistant who answered all my questions during the recovery period, like 'when will my bruises go away?' and 'when can I drive again?'" Richardson notes.

Adjusting to Change

Like most women who undergo reduction, Mary-Margaret Richardson, Kellie Feldman, and Margie were pleased with the results. "Of all the procedures I do, this one has the highest patient satisfaction, even when the results are less than perfect," Beraka says.

"I'm amazed whenever I go shopping. I can buy a dress, not separates with the top four sizes larger. My posture is so much better, and there's no rutting in my shoulders. Most of all, the pain in my neck and back is gone," Richardson says.

"I no longer have rashes under my breasts or shoulder indentations," Feldman adds. "Plus, I went on a diet and lost a total of 28 pounds, seven of which was breast tissue. I feel much healthier."

"People ask, 'why did you wait so long?'" Richardson notes. "I tell them that when it began to be debilitating, everything sort of came together. I was scared up until the night before the surgery. But the time was right. I don't regret one minute of it."

—by Marilyn Larkin

Chapter 31

Gynecomastia— Correction of Enlarged Male Breasts

A Word about Breast Reduction in Men

Gynecomastia is a medical term that comes from the Greek words for "women-like breasts." Though this oddly named condition is rarely talked about, it's actually quite common. Gynecomastia affects an estimated 40 to 60 percent of men. It may affect only one breast or both. Though certain drugs and medical problems have been linked with male breast over-development, there is no known cause in the vast majority of cases.

For men who feel self-conscious about their appearance, breast-reduction surgery can help. The procedure removes fat and or glandular tissue from the breasts, and in extreme cases removes excess skin, resulting in a chest that is flatter, firmer, and better contoured.

If you're considering surgery to correct gynecomastia, this chapter will give you a basic understanding of the procedure—when it can help, how it's performed, and what results you can expect. It can't answer all of your questions, since a lot depends on your individual circumstances. Please be sure to ask your doctor if there is anything about the procedure you don't understand.

American Society of Plastic Surgeons, reprinted from The Plastic Surgery Information Service at www.plasticsurgery.org. © 1994; reprinted with permission.

The Best Candidates for Gynecomastia Correction

Surgery to correct gynecomastia can be performed on healthy, emotionally stable men of any age. The best candidates for surgery have firm, elastic skin that will reshape to the body's new contours.

Surgery may be discouraged for obese men, or for overweight men who have not first attempted to correct the problem with exercise or weight loss. Also, individuals who drink alcohol beverages in excess or smoke marijuana are usually not considered good candidates for surgery. These drugs, along with anabolic steroids, may cause gynecomastia. Therefore, patients are first directed to stop the use of these drugs to see if the breast fullness will diminish before surgery is considered an option.

All Surgery Carries Some Uncertainty and Risk

When male breast-reduction surgery is performed by a qualified plastic surgeon, complications are infrequent and usually minor. Nevertheless, as with any surgery, there are risks. These include infection, skin injury, excessive bleeding, adverse reaction to anesthesia, and excessive fluid loss or accumulation. The procedure may also result in noticeable scars, permanent pigment changes in the breast area, or slightly mismatched breasts or nipples. If asymmetry is significant, a second procedure may be performed to remove additional tissue. The temporary effects of breast reduction include loss of breast sensation or numbness, which may last up to a year.

Planning Your Surgery

The initial consultation with your surgeon is very important. Your surgeon will need a complete medical history, so check your own records ahead of time and be ready to provide this information. First, your surgeon will examine your breasts and check for causes of the gynecomastia, such as impaired liver function, use of estrogen-containing medications, or anabolic steroids. If a medical problem is the suspected cause, you'll be referred to an appropriate specialist.

Your plastic surgeon may, in extreme cases, also recommend a mammogram, or breast x-ray. This will not only rule out the very small possibility of breast cancer, but will reveal the breast's composition. Once your surgeon knows how much fat and glandular tissue is contained within the breasts, he or she can choose a surgical approach to best suit your needs.

Don't hesitate to ask your surgeon any questions you may have during the initial consultation—including your concerns about the recommended treatment or the costs involved. Treatment of gynecomastia may be covered by medical insurance—but policies vary greatly. Check your policy or call your carrier to be sure. If you are covered, make certain you get written pre-authorization for the treatment recommended by your surgeon.

Preparing for Your Surgery

Your surgeon will give you specific instructions on how to prepare for surgery, including guidelines on eating, drinking, and taking certain vitamins and medications.

Smokers should plan to stop smoking for a minimum of one or two weeks before surgery and during recovery. Smoking decreases circulation and interferes with proper healing. Therefore, it is essential to follow all your surgeon's instructions.

Where Your Surgery Will be Performed

Surgery for gynecomastia is most often performed as an outpatient procedure, but in extreme cases, or those where other medical conditions present cause for concern, an overnight hospital stay may be recommended. The surgery itself usually takes about an hour and a half to complete. However, more extensive procedures may take longer.

Type of Anesthesia

Correction of enlarged male breasts may be performed under general, or in some cases, under local anesthesia plus sedation. You'll be awake, but very relaxed and insensitive to pain. More extensive correction may be performed under general anesthesia, which allows the patient to sleep through the entire operation. Your surgeon will discuss which option is recommended for you, and why this is the option of choice.

The Surgery

If excess glandular tissue is the primary cause of the breast enlargement, it will be excised, or cut out, with a scalpel. The excision may be performed alone or in conjunction with liposuction. In a typical procedure, an incision is made in an inconspicuous location—either on the edge of the areola or in the underarm area. Working through the incision, the surgeon cuts away the excess glandular tissue, fat and skin from around the areola and from the sides and bottom of the breast. Major reductions that involve the removal of a significant amount of tissue and skin may require larger incisions that result in more conspicuous scars. If liposuction is used to remove excess fat, the cannula is usually inserted through the existing incisions.

If your gynecomastia consists primarily of excessive fatty tissue, your surgeon will likely use liposuction to remove the excess fat. A small incision, less than a half-inch in length, is made around the edge of the areola—the dark skin that surrounds the nipple. Or, the incision may be placed in the underarm area. A slim hollow tube called a cannula which is attached to a vacuum pump, is then inserted into the incision. Using strong, deliberate strokes, the surgeon moves the cannula through the layers beneath the skin, breaking up the fat and suctioning it out. Patients may feel a vibration or some friction during the procedure, but generally no pain.

In extreme cases where large amounts of fat or glandular tissue have been removed, skin may not adjust well to the new smaller breast contour. In these cases, excess skin may have to be removed to allow the removing skin to firmly readjust to the new breast contour.

Sometimes, a small drain is inserted through a separate incision to draw off excess fluids. Once closed, the incisions are usually covered with a dressing. The chest may be wrapped to keep the skin firmly in place.

After Your Surgery

Whether you've had excision with a scalpel or liposuction, you will feel some discomfort for a few days after surgery. However, discomfort can be controlled with medications prescribed by your surgeon. In any case, you should arrange to have someone drive you home after surgery and to help you out for a day or two if needed.

You'll be swollen and bruised for awhile—in fact, you may wonder if there's been any improvement at all. To help reduce swelling, you'll probably be instructed to wear an elastic pressure garment continuously for a week or two, and for a few weeks longer at night. Although the worst of your swelling will dissipate in the first few weeks, it may be three months or more before the final results of your surgery are apparent.

In the meantime, it is important to begin getting back to normal. You'll be encouraged to begin walking around on the day of surgery, and can return to work when you feel well enough—which could be as early as a day or two after surgery. Any stitches will generally be removed about one to two weeks following the procedure.

Your surgeon may advise you to avoid sexual activity for a week or two, and heavy exercise for about three weeks. You'll be told to stay away from any sport or job that risks a blow to the chest area for at least four weeks. In general, it will take about a month before you're back to all of your normal activities.

You should also avoid exposing the resulting scars to the sun for at least six months. Sunlight can permanently affect the skin's pigmentation, causing the scar to turn dark. If sun exposure is unavoidable, use a strong sun block.

Your New Look

Gynecomastia surgery can enhance your appearance and self-confidence, but it won't necessarily change your looks to match your ideal. Before you decide to have surgery, think carefully about your expectations and discuss them frankly with your plastic surgeon.

The results of the procedure are significant and permanent. If your expectations are realistic, chances are good that you'll be very satisfied with your new look.

Additional information on plastic surgery is available from the Plastic Surgery Information Service web site at www.plasticsurgery.org or call (800) 635-0635.

Chapter 32

Tumescent Liposuction

Liposuction was first developed in the late 1970s to remove undesired fat from nearly all body areas, including the face, neck, chin, breast, abdomen, hips, flanks (love handles), inner and outer thighs, buttocks, knees, and ankles. Developed by dermatologic surgeons in the 1980s, a major advancement called the tumescent technique of liposuction completely revolutionized the procedure. The use of tumescent liposuction allows dermatologic surgeons to safely and effectively remove deep and superficial layers of fat under local anesthesia with relatively little discomfort, virtually no complications and improved cosmetic results.

What Is Liposuction?

Liposuction is the removal of excess fat with a small, straw-like instrument called a cannula that is attached to a suction machine. The fat layer under the skin is converted to a network of tunnels, and the cannula is manipulated within the layers to remove unwanted fatty deposits. An elastic garment is then worn for compression and healing. The result is a resculpting of bulging areas into more attractive contours.

When Is Liposuction Indicated?

Liposuction is most effective for removing localized fat deposits in body areas that do not respond to dieting or exercising. Liposuction

American Society for Dermatologic Surgery, Form No. 003, 1994. © 1995-1999; reprinted with permission.

155

is not intended as a substitute for weight loss, but rather is a contouring procedure. It is best utilized in a program of exercise and optimal weight maintenance. Liposuction also has many valuable therapeutic applications and has been used effectively to treat medical conditions like excessive sweating and non-cosmetic fat accumulation, such as lipomas (benign fatty tumors) and gynecomastia (enlarged, male breasts).

What Happens Prior to Surgery?

Before surgery, a complete medical history is taken and a careful examination is conducted in order to evaluate your condition. During the consultation, your dermatologic surgeon describes the procedure and what results might realistically be expected. Your doctor also will review alternative treatment options and explain the possible risks and complications that may occur. Photographs are frequently taken before and after surgery to help evaluate the amount of improvement.

How Is the Tumescent Technique of Liposuction Performed?

Liposuction can be performed in the dermatologic surgeon's office facility, in an outpatient surgical suite or in a hospital. If general anesthesia is not otherwise indicated, its potential complications can be avoided by the use of local anesthesia (often used with light sedation) via the tumescent technique. This breakthrough technique refers to filling the skin with local anesthetic in order to remove unwanted fat more efficiently.

With tumescent liposuction, large volumes of a solution containing dilute lidocaine (a local anesthetic) and dilute epinephrine (a drug to shrink capillaries and prevent blood loss) are injected with minimal discomfort directly into areas of excessive fatty deposits. Once the liquid is injected, a small incision is made in the skin, and a tube connected to a vacuum is inserted into the fatty layer. Using to and fro movements, the fat is drawn through the tube into a collection system. The tumescent method enables the dermatologic surgeon to remove large amounts of fat more uniformly with fewer skin irregularities and less bleeding and bruising.

What Happens after Surgery?

The local anesthesia injected into the tissue remains for 18 to 24 hours following liposuction surgery, greatly minimizing postoperative pain. After tumescent liposuction, patients are usually alert and able to function without nausea, grogginess and the "washed out" feeling associated with general anesthesia. With the tumescent technique, there is minimal bruising, and many patients do not require postoperative medication for pain. You can usually return to a desk-type job within 48 hours; physical exercise generally can be resumed three to seven days after liposuction.

Are There Any Possible Complications?

The tumescent technique of liposuction is a remarkably safe procedure with few significant side effects. A recent study in the *Dermatologic Surgery Journal* reported that 112 patients who underwent the tumescent procedure had an average of two quarts of fat removed with no significant complications. Clinical studies by other specialists have also demonstrated the safety and efficacy of tumescent liposuction.

What Are the Limitations of Liposuction?

Liposuction is not intended as a method for weight loss. It is used as a shaping procedure for areas where hereditary fat deposits resistant to diet and exercise have accumulated. The best results from liposuction occur in body areas where there is reasonable muscle tone, where skin has good elastic quality, and where fat is not excessive. In cases where there is a significant loss of tone and elasticity, superior cosmetic results may require a combination of both liposuction and surgical skin tightening to remove the excessive loose tissue.

Your dermatologic surgeon can advise you of the likelihood of the need for additional treatments, depending on the specific condition of your skin.

What Is Ultrasonic Liposuction?

Another advance in tumescent liposuction is the use of internal or external ultrasound. The ultrasonic method introduces high-frequency sound waves and mechanical vibrations with a hand-held cannula placed into or on top of skin or fatty tissue to gently break down and liquefy the fat cells prior to liposuctioning. The fat is then removed via tumescent liposuction under local anesthesia. Potential advantages to this approach include the ability to remove fat in difficult areas such as the upper abdomen, the flanks, the back, and the male chest.

For More Information

For more information on skin conditions and liposuction treatment, along with a referral list of dermatologic surgeons in specific geographic areas, please call the ASDS toll-free hotline, 1-800-441-2737, during weekday business hours (CST) or visit our Web site at http://www.asds-net.org/.

American Society for Dermatologic Surgery (ASDS)

The ASDS provides continuing training and education for its members in new dermatologic surgical techniques and procedures. Represented in the American Medical Association House of Delegates, the ASDS was formed in 1970 to promote the highest standards of patient care for the surgical treatment of the skin, hair, nails, veins, and mucous membranes.

Chapter 33

Tummy Tuck (Abdominoplasty)

The tummy tuck is an operation that is designed to remove excess skin from the abdomen at the same time, tightening the abdominal muscles. It is indicated in cases where there is laxity of the abdomen resulting in bulging due to abnormal stretching of the abdominal muscles and skin. Unlike liposuction surgery, which just removes fat, this operation involves removal of skin and fat, with tightening of the abdominal muscles. For this reason, it is more extensive than liposuction. The actual extent of surgery will depend on the amount of excess skin and the laxity of the abdominal muscles.

In some cases, liposuction surgery can be combined with excision of excess abdominal skin instead of a more complete tummy tuck. Although this does not give as good a skin tightening, it does result in much smaller scars and a shorter recovery period. When a full tummy tuck is contemplated, however, extensive liposuction is best delayed until a later time, since there seems to be a higher chance of complications when the two procedures are combined. Not uncommonly, touch-up liposuction is done under local anesthesia after the original operation.

For patients with bulging muscle and excess fat, whose skin is relatively tight, an endoscopic abdominoplasty is an option that is rapidly gaining popularity. It is discussed below.

Howard A. Tobin, M.D., F.A.C.S., Facial Plastic & Cosmetic Surgical Center, reprinted from the website at www.newlook.com. © 2000; reprinted with permission.

159

Prior to tummy tuck surgery, the amount of skin that is to be removed is carefully marked. The operation is carried out under general anesthesia. An incision is made in the bikini line and the excess skin is pulled down and inward, and is removed along with underlying fatty tissue. The muscles are tightened as required, the skin is carefully re-draped and the incision closed with several layers of suture. In most cases, the belly button will have to be repositioned because of the amount of skin removed. Contrary to what you may think, the belly button is not removed during the operation!

Following surgery, a compressive girdle and stockings are worn for a few weeks. There may be considerable discomfort for several days following surgery but most patients resume limited activity in a day or so. A urinary catheter is normally left in place for several hours after surgery, and wound drains are kept in place for a few days to help prevent the accumulation of fluid. Because of the risk of possible pulmonary emboli or partial lung collapse, it is important for patients to begin movement promptly after surgery, even if it is uncomfortable.

Because of the extent of the surgery, there are risks involved which can result in serious complications. Infection or collections of blood or fluid in the wound may delay recovery and could result in skin loss, fat necrosis or scarring. These could lead to the need for additional corrective surgery. The abdominal wall is stretched during surgery and the blood supply to the skin may be damaged. This may lead to loss of skin. If this happens a skin graft may be needed if the wound does not heal, although usually, in these circumstances primary healing will occur, though it could take months.

Fortunately, most tummy tucks are uncomplicated, but patients must be prepared for the added time needed for recovery when complications occur. In addition, patients must realize that there is a sizable scar, which, although hidden, may thicken or widen requiring later revision. It is also important to realize that it will take many months for the scar to fade to its final appearance. Unfortunately, because of the pull involved with the operation, it is not uncommon for scars to be somewhat widened or irregular. About 20 percent of patients will return after about one year for scar revision.

In spite of these considerations, the operation is generally very gratifying. Many patients realize relief of functional symptoms such as low back pain, rash and abdominal discomfort following the surgery. When surgery is primarily sought for functional purposes, insurance may help cover the cost. If you feel that your condition fits these criteria, consult your medical staff who can help you to obtain that information from your insurance company.

Tummy tucks are often carried out in an outpatient surgical center; however, some patients will require hospitalization, especially for the more extensive procedures. If patients choose to have surgery on an outpatient basis, they must understand that if any complications develop, hospitalization may be required and could involve additional cost, which may not be covered by insurance. Although a more major procedure than liposuction surgery, in many cases, abdominoplasty will provide the type of contour improvement that patients are seeking, which cannot be provided by other means.

While abdominoplasty remains a popular option for women with excess abdominal skin and fat combined with muscular laxity, admittedly it is an extensive surgical procedure. Patients must be prepared for a few weeks of recovery and be willing to accept a long scar that is a necessary part of the surgical procedure.

Certainly, many patients who formerly considered abdominoplasty now obtain satisfactory results from liposuction surgery alone, but fat suctioning does nothing to tighten up the abdominal muscles. A gap has existed between candidates for liposuction surgery alone and those who need either a full abdominoplasty or abdominoplasty combined with liposuction surgery. The endoscopic abdominoplasty is filling this gap. The operation involves a tightening of the abdominal muscles through an endoscopic approach.

Like all endoscopic procedures, this type of abdominoplasty can really be considered Band-Aid surgery. Working entirely through tiny incisions often limited to a single incision around the belly button, we can tighten up the abdominal muscles by suturing with special instruments, while viewing through telescopes and cameras that are designed for the job. Laser surgery can be used to assist the dissection. It is applicable for patients with moderate to mild muscle bulging, primarily in patients who have not had previous major surgery of the abdomen.

Endoscopic abdominoplasty is an exciting new horizon in cosmetic surgery. Recovery is generally very prompt. In fact most patients resume relatively normal activity within a few days. Discomfort is somewhat more than liposuction alone, but usually does not interfere with normal activity after a week or so. Surgical drains are required for a few days to prevent accumulation of fluid that can sometimes occur. If fluid builds up after the drains are removed, it may require removal by aspiration with a syringe. At the time of this writing we have seen few other complications, although bleeding and infection are possible. During your consultation we will review any additional risks or complications that may have arisen.

As with all endoscopic cosmetic surgery, this is a new field, and techniques and instrumentation are continuing to evolve. We anticipate that there will be new applications for this type of procedure. Our experience with the endoscopic abdominoplasty has been very favorable, and it is an operation that is gaining popularity.

For additional information contact: Howard A. Tobin, M.D., F.A.C.S., Facial Plastic & Cosmetic Surgical Center, 6300 Regional Plaza, Abilene, Texas 79606. (915) 695-3630; Toll Free (800) 592-4533; Fax (915) 695-3633; e-mail: n41gt@newlook.com.

Chapter 34

Treatments for Spider and Varicose Veins

Why are Spider and Varicose Veins a Concern?

Varicose and smaller spider veins affect an estimated 80 million adults in the United States. Even shapely legs can look less attractive with bulging blue veins or a network of spider veins. In fact, a recent survey indicated that American women are more concerned about leg veins than almost any other cosmetic problem.

The exact cause of spider and varicose veins is unknown, although heredity, pregnancy and hormonal changes are believed to be contributing factors. As people age, these unsightly veins become more common and often more pronounced. Forty-one percent of women aged 40-50 years old have varicose veins, increasing to 72 percent of women aged 60-70 years old. Among men aged 30-40 years old, 24 percent have varicose veins, increasing to 43 percent among 70-year-old men.

While usually a cosmetic condition, varicose veins may also pose a health risk. In fact, six million workdays each year are lost due to complications from varicose veins. The abnormal circulation resulting from varicose veins may cause ulcers, and it is estimated that nearly 100,000 Americans are totally disabled by the condition.

What are Spider and Varicose Veins?

Spider veins are formed by the dilation of a small group of blood vessels located close to the surface of the skin. Although they can

American Society for Dermatologic Surgery, Form No. 009, 1998, © 1995-1999; reprinted with permission.

appear anywhere on the body, spider veins are most commonly found on the face and legs and look like red or purple sunbursts or web patterns. Spider veins are also referred to as telangiectasia or broken capillaries. They usually pose no health hazard but may produce a dull aching in the legs after prolonged standing.

Varicose veins are swollen or enlarged blood vessels caused by a weakening in the vein's wall or valves. They are located somewhat deeper than spider veins, are sometimes raised, and often appear blue. The origin of these varicose veins may be hidden under the skin. Advanced cases of varicose veins can be harmful to a patient's health because they may be associated with the development of one or more of the following conditions:

- Venous stasis ulcers, which can result when the enlarged vein does not provide adequate drainage of fluid from the skin. The swollen skin receives insufficient oxygen and an ulcer forms.

- Phlebitis, which is an inflammation of the vein.

- Thromboses, which are blood clots forming in the enlarged vein.

Who is Qualified to Treat Spider and Varicose Veins?

Dermatologic surgeons have extensive training and experience in the diagnosis and treatment of vein disorders. As specialists in diseases of the skin, dermatologic surgeons are uniquely qualified to select the treatment method or combination of methods that works best in a particular situation and provides the optimal cosmetic results.

How Are Veins Treated?

A number of surgical treatment options are used to improve vein conditions. All treatments are intended to remove or destroy a defective vein so that its function can be quickly taken over by healthy veins. In most cases, leg compression is recommended with one or more treatment method.

Sclerotherapy

Sclerotherapy is a safe and effective procedure that can be performed by a dermatologic surgeon in the doctor's office with minimal discomfort. A concentrated saline or specially developed chemical solution is injected with a very small needle into the spider or varicose vein. The sclerosing (hardening) solution causes the vein to close up or collapse and become scar tissue that eventually is absorbed by the body. The work of carrying the blood is shifted to other healthy blood vessels nearby.

Sclerotherapy generally requires multiple treatment sessions. One to three injection sessions are usually required to effectively treat any vein, and 10 to 40 veins may be treated in one session. The same area should not be retreated for four to six weeks to allow for complete healing, although other areas may undergo treatment during this time. Occasionally diagnostic tests such as ultrasound or plethysmography may be recommended to enhance the results of treatment.

Post-treatment therapy includes wearing compression bandages or support hose for two days to three weeks following treatment. Walking and moderate exercise may also help speed recovery. The treated blood vessels generally disappear over a period of six months. Although sclerotherapy works for existing spider veins, it does not prevent new ones from developing.

Are There Any Side Effects Following Treatment?

Most patients report few, if any minor side effects from sclerotherapy, which usually disappear in time. Temporary reactions can include a slight swelling of the leg or foot, minor bruising, itching, redness, a small erosion, or moderate soreness. Rarely, a scar may result.

What Other Treatments Are Used for Spider and Varicose Veins?

Ambulatory Phlebectomy: This technique involves removal of an undesired vein through a series of tiny punctures or incisions along the path of the enlarged vein. Using a specially designed instrument to "hook" the varicose vein into the dermatologic surgeon's view, the damaged vein can be removed entirely by gently pulling from tiny puncture to puncture. This safe, outpatient procedure can treat large varicose veins, as well as small spider veins, with minimal risks, reduced side effects, and decreased recurrence.

Electrodesiccation: The veins are sealed off with the application of electrical current.

Laser surgery and intense pulsed light therapy: This relatively new approach may be effective for certain leg veins and facial blood vessels. The heat from the high intensity laser beam or intense pulsed light device selectively destroys the abnormal veins.

Surgical ligation and stripping: This method involves making an incision in the skin and either tying off or removing the blood vessel. The procedure may require the use of general anesthesia, is usually performed by a vascular surgeon in the hospital, and is generally reserved for larger veins.

For More Information

For more information on the treatment of vein conditions and to obtain a referral list of dermatologic surgeons offering treatment in your geographic area, call the American Society for Dermatologic Surgery's toll-free consumer hotline, 1-800-441-2737, during weekday business hours (CST), or visit their Web site at www.asds-net.org.

The American Society for Dermatologic Surgery (ASDS)

The ASDS provides grants, training and continuing education for its members in new dermatologic surgical techniques and procedures. Represented in the American Medical Association House of Delegates, the Society was formed in 1970 to promote excellence in the subspecialty of dermatologic surgery and to foster the highest standards of patient care.

Part Five

Reconstructive Plastic Surgery

Chapter 35

Cleft Lip and Palate Surgery

If You're Considering Surgery to Correct Cleft Lip or Palate

In the early weeks of development, long before a child is born, the right and left sides of the lip and the roof of the mouth normally grow together. Occasionally, however, in about one of every 800 babies, those sections don't quite meet. A child born with a separation in the upper lip is said to have a cleft lip. A similar birth defect in the roof of the mouth, or palate, is called a cleft palate. Since the lip and the palate develop separately, it is possible for a child to have a cleft lip, a cleft palate, or variations of both.

If your child was born with either or both of these conditions, your doctor will probably recommend surgery to repair it. Medical professionals have made great advances in treating children with clefts and can do a lot to help your child lead a normal, healthy, happy life.

This information will give you a basic understanding of the operation—when it can help, how it's performed, and what results you can expect. It can't answer all of your questions, since a lot depends on you individual circumstances. Please be sure to ask your surgeon if there is anything you don't understand about the procedure.

American Society of Plastic Surgeons, reprinted from The Plastic Surgery Information Service at www.plasticsurgery.org. © 1992; reprinted with permission.

The Importance of a Team Approach

Children born with a cleft lip or palate may need the skills of several medical professionals to correct the problems associated with the cleft. In addition to needing plastic surgery to repair the opening, these children may have problems with their feeding and their teeth, their hearing, their speech, and their psychological development as they grow up.

For that reason, parents should seek the help of a Cleft Lip and Palate Team as early as possible. Medical professionals with special experience in the problems of cleft lip and palate have formed such teams all over the country to help parents plan for their child's care from birth, or even before. Typically, a Cleft Team might include a plastic surgeon, a pediatrician, a dentist, a speech and language specialist, a social worker, a hearing specialist, an ear-nose-throat specialist, a psychologist, a nurse, and a genetic counselor.

Ask your doctor for a referral to a Cleft Team in your area. Or, for more information, contact The Cleft Palate Foundation, 1218 Grandview Avenue, Pittsburgh, PA, 15211; (412) 481-1376.

All Surgery Carries Some Uncertainty and Risk

When surgery is done by a qualified plastic surgeon with experience in repairing cleft lip or palate, the results can be quite positive. Nevertheless, as with any operation, there are risks associated with surgery and specific complications associated with this procedure.

In cleft lip surgery, the most common problem is asymmetry, when one side of the mouth and nose does not match the other side. The goal of cleft lip surgery is to close the separation in the first operation. Occasionally, a second operation may be needed.

In cleft palate surgery, the goal is to close the opening in the roof of the mouth so the child can eat and learn to speak properly. Occasionally, poor healing in the palate or poor speech may require a second operation.

Planning for Surgery

At your initial consultation, your doctor will discuss the details of the procedure he or she will use, including where the surgery will be performed, the type of anesthesia to be used, possible risks and complications, recovery, costs, and the results you can expect. Your surgeon will also answer any questions you may have about feeding your baby, by breast or by bottle, both before and after the surgery.

In most cases, health insurance policies will cover most or all of the cost of cleft lip or cleft palate surgery. Check your policy to make sure your child is covered and to see if there are any limitations on what types of treatment are covered.

Cleft Lip Surgery

A cleft lip can range in severity from a slight notch in the red part of the upper lip to a complete separation of the lip extending into the nose. Clefts can occur on one or both sides of the upper lip. Surgery is generally done when the child is about 10 weeks old.

To repair a cleft lip, the surgeon will make an incision on either side of the cleft from the mouth into the nostril. He or she will then turn the dark pink outer portion of the cleft down and pull the muscle and the skin of the lip together to close the separation. Muscle function and the normal "cupid's bow" shape of the mouth are restored. The nostril deformity often associated with cleft lip may also be improved at the time of lip repair or in a later surgery.

Recovering from Cleft Lip Surgery

Your child may be restless for awhile after surgery, but your doctor can prescribe medication to relieve any discomfort. Elbow restraints may be necessary for a few weeks to prevent your baby from rubbing the stitched area.

If dressings have been used, they'll be removed within a day or two, and the stitches will either dissolve or be removed within five days. Your doctor will advise you on how to feed your child during the first few weeks after surgery.

It's normal for the surgical scar to appear to get bigger and redder for a few weeks after surgery. This will gradually fade, although the scar will never totally disappear. In many children, however, it's barely noticeable because of the shadows formed by the nose and upper lip.

Cleft Palate Surgery

In some children, a cleft palate may involve only a tiny portion at the back of the roof of the mouth; for others, it can mean a complete separation that extends from front to back. Just as in cleft lip, cleft palate may appear on one or both sides of the upper mouth. However, repairing a cleft palate involves more extensive surgery and is usually done when the child is nine to 18 months old, so the baby is bigger and better able to tolerate surgery.

To repair a cleft palate, the surgeon will make an incision on both sides of the separation, moving tissue from each side of the cleft to the center or midline of the roof of the mouth. This rebuilds the palate, joining muscle together and providing enough length in the palate so the child can eat and learn to speak properly.

Recovering from Cleft Palate Surgery

For a day or two, your child will probably feel some soreness and pain, which is easily controlled by medication. During this period, you child will not eat or drink as much as usual—so an intravenous line will be used to maintain fluid levels. Elbow restraints may be used to prevent your baby from rubbing the repaired area. Your doctor will advise you on how to feed your child during the first few weeks after surgery. It's crucial that you follow your doctor's advice on feeding to allow the palate to heal properly.

The Repaired Lip or Palate

Children with a cleft palate are particularly prone to ear infections because the cleft can interfere with the function of the middle ear. To permit proper drainage and air circulation, the ear-nose-and-throat surgeon on the Cleft Palate Team may recommend that a small plastic ventilation tube be inserted in the eardrum. This relatively minor operation may be done later or at the time of the cleft repair. In addition, surgery may be recommended by your plastic surgeon when your child is older to refine the shape and function of the lip, nose, gums, and palate. You'll want to discuss further needs with the members of the Cleft Team seeing your child.

Perhaps most important, keep in mind that surgery to repair a cleft lip or palate is only the beginning of the process. Family support is critical for your child. Love and understanding will help him or her grow up with a sense of self-esteem that extends beyond the physical defect.

Additional information on plastic surgery is available from the Plastic Surgery Information Service web site at www.plasticsurgery.org or call (800) 635-0635.

Chapter 36

Septoplasty

What Is a Septoplasty?

A septoplasty is a surgical procedure in which the nasal septum is straightened.

What Is the Nasal Septum?

The nasal septum is the part of the nose that divides the right nasal cavity from the left nasal cavity (see diagrams). The septum usually lies directly in the center of the nose and rests on a bony ridge called the maxillary crest. The septum is made up of several layers. In the front, the central portion of the septum is cartilage, a relatively soft material that is fairly flexible. More posteriorly, the central septum is made up of thin bone. Lying on top of the bone and cartilage is the lining of the nose, called the mucosa.

When and Why Is a Septoplasty Done?

A septoplasty is done if the septum is so crooked that it interferes with breathing or causes other problems. Few people actually have a perfectly straight septum, but in most cases the amount of bending is not large enough to be noticed.

The Voice Center of Eastern Virginia Medical School, Norfolk, VA. Reprinted from www.voice-center.com. © 1999; reprinted with permission.

The most common symptom from a badly deviated (crooked) septum is difficult breathing through the nose. The symptoms are usually worse on one side, and sometimes actually occur on the side opposite the bend. In some cases the crooked septum can interfere with the drainage of the sinuses, resulting in repeated sinus infections. The septum may also need to be straightened in individuals undergoing sinus surgery, just so that the instruments needed for this operation can be fit into the nasal cavity.

I Have Stuffy Breathing. Does this Mean I Need a Septoplasty?

It is important to remember that the nose goes through a natural cycle in which the nasal line on one side and then the other slowly expands and contracts. These cycles occur every several hours and may lead to the perception of nasal obstruction. If you have persistent difficult breathing through your nose, you should see an Otolaryngologist for a complete exam.

Should I Use Nasal Sprays to Improve Breathing Through My Nose?

You should NOT use any over-the-counter nasal sprays for more than a few days without contacting your doctor. Many of these products have ingredients that produce rebound nasal swelling when they are stopped. As a result, the user is required to keep using the spray in order to keep his or her nose clear. Long-term use like this can cause injury to the lining of the nose. There are some sprays that can be used for a long time without side effects; ask your doctor which spray is best for you.

How Is a Septoplasty Done?

The basic principle in a septoplasty is to straighten the crooked portions of the septum. The operation is almost always done through the nose, without an external incision (there may be an incision if a rhinoplasty is also done at the same time). Badly deviated portions of the septum may be removed entirely, or they may be removed, readjusted, and reinserted into the nose.

The operation takes about one to one-and-one-half hours, depending on the complexity of the deviation. It can be done with a local or a general anesthetic, and is usually done on an outpatient basis. In many cases nasal packing is placed for one to several days. There almost never is any bruising on the skin for just a septoplasty, though there can be bruising if a rhinoplasty is also done at the same time.

What Are the Potential Complications of a Septoplasty?

If the operation is done under a general anesthetic, there are the usual risks associated with any general anesthesia. Bleeding is a possible risk, which may require nasal packing. Much more rare is the risk of a hole developing in the septum after the operation. This may cause nasal crusting or interfere with breathing through the nose. An even rarer complication is postoperative infection of the septum, which could cause the front portion of the nose to bend inward. This would require a second operation to correct the deformity.

How Do I Know If I Need a Septoplasty?

It is best to have a good nasal exam by an Otolaryngologist. There are some medical treatments that can reduce nasal swelling and eliminate the need for nasal surgery.

Chapter 37

Surgical Treatments for Craniofacial Syndromes

Contents

Section 37.1

Down Syndrome

World Craniofacial Foundation, reprinted from their website at
www.worldcf.org. © 1998; reprinted with permission.

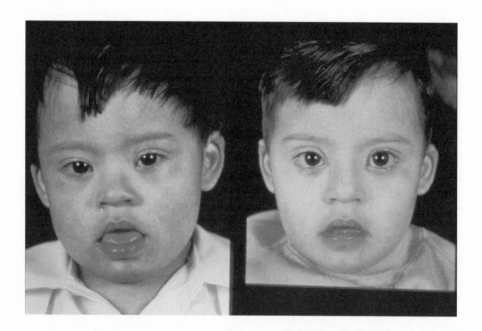

Figure 37.1. *Down Syndrome patient before and after surgery.*

Down Syndrome, also known as Trisomy 21 due to the presence of
a third twenty-first chromosome, is one of the most common and well
known birth anomalies. One in every 650 children born will be affected
by this syndrome.

Characteristics

Some of the facial features which identify an individual as having Down Syndrome include:

- Low set ears,
- Up slanting palpebral fissures,
- Low nasal bridge and dorsum,
- Abnormal and excessive facial fat distribution, and
- Protruding, enlarged tongue.

Expectations

Both prenatal and postnatal growth deficiencies can exist in the Down patients. They often exhibit a short stocky stature and also have delayed growth of the brain resulting in a reduced mental capacity. The extent to which they are intellectually deficient varies from patient to patient. Although there have been many advances in the medical care of these patients, the life expectancy of a patient with Down Syndrome is 35 years of age.

Treatment

Although the craniofacial manifestations of this syndrome may not be medically threatening, the psychological aspect of these anomalies can be harmful. Due to the similar appearance of those with this syndrome, they tend to resemble each other rather then their respective families. With this in mind, the goal of the reconstruction of these malformations is to increase the resemblance of these patients to their families.

Treatment of the anomalies associated with this syndrome include a surgery to correct the eye slant and to remove the skin folds from the inner corners of the eyes. These patients usually require nasal surgery to augment and increase the projection of their nose. In addition, some of the fat in their cheek can be removed to reduce the fullness of their face. It may also be necessary to reduce the size of their tongue to increase its mobility and improve their speech.

Section 37.2

Goldenhar Syndrome

World Craniofacial Foundation, reprinted from their website at
www.worldcf.org. © 1998; reprinted with permission.

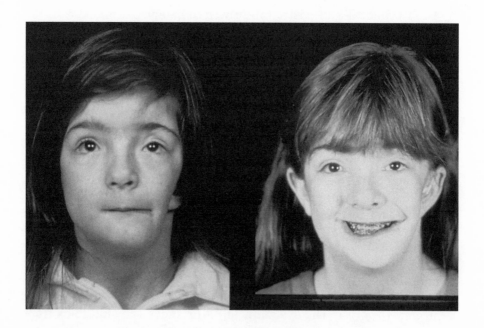

***Figure 37.2.** Goldenhar Syndrome patient before and after surgery.*

Goldenhar Syndrome is a variant of Hemifacial Microsomia. Its
severity can vary and the effects can be unilateral or bilateral. The
physical manifestations of this disorder match those of hemifacial
microsomia with the addition of epibulbar dermoids which are benign
tumors located just inside the opening of the eye or the eyeballs.

Characteristics

The physical characteristics of Goldenhar Syndrome include:

- Unilateral or bilateral underdevelopment of the mandible,

- Unilateral or bilateral microtia,

- Unilateral or bilateral reduction in size and flattening of the maxilla (upper jaw),

- Narrowing of the opening of the eye, and

- Epibulbar Dermoids which can cause problems with vision.

The lack of growth and facial asymmetry of Hemifacial Microsomia are accompanied by epibulbar dermoids.

Expectations

Due to the delayed growth and development of the affected areas, the effects of this syndrome will be more evident as the child grows. The lack of the development of the upper and lower jaws can cause breathing problems as well as a dental malocclusion which will need to be addressed surgically and orthodontically.

Treatment

For these patients, treatment generally requires the expertise of both a craniofacial surgeon and an orthodontist with experience with these problems. The jaw deformity is addressed as early as three years of age if the mandibular retrusion is severe enough to cause airway difficulty. This jaw reconstruction can be achieved by extending the mandible with a rib graft or with the utilization of a distraction device to "stretch" the bone. The best approach to reconstructing the jaw is determined by the surgeon and is specific for each patient. If it is needed, ear reconstruction is performed in four stages and usually begins at the age of six years. Throughout life, these patients must maintain adequate dental occlusion through ongoing orthodontic treatment.

Information on this page is from: World Craniofacial Foundation, reprinted from their website at www.worldcf.org. © 1998; reprinted with permission.

Section 37.3

Hemifacial Microsomia

World Craniofacial Foundation, reprinted from their website at
www.worldcf.org. © 1998; reprinted with permission.

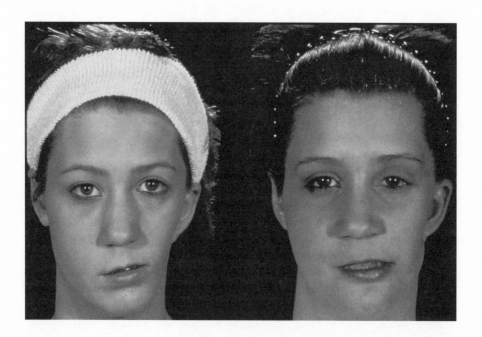

Figure 37.3. *Hemifacial microsomia patient before and after surgery.*

Hemifacial microsomia is a condition that affects the growth of the
face unilaterally or bilaterally. The severity of this disorder can vary
from mild to severe. Although different facial structures can be affected, the most common areas include the ear, the oral cavity, and
the mandible.

Characteristics

The physical features of hemifacial microsomia include the following:

- Unilateral or bilateral underdevelopment of the mandible (lower jaw),

- Unilateral or bilateral underdevelopment of the ear,

- Unilateral or bilateral reduction in size and flattening of the maxilla (upper jaw), and

- Narrowing of the opening of the eye.

Expectations

Due to the delayed growth and development of the affected areas, the effects of this syndrome will be more evident as the child grows. The lack of the development of the upper and lower jaws can cause breathing problems, as well as a dental malocclusion which will need to be addressed surgically and orthodontically.

Treatment

For these patients, treatment generally requires the expertise of both a craniofacial surgeon and an orthodontist with experience with these problems. The jaw deformity is addressed as early as three years of age if the mandibular retrusion is severe enough to cause airway difficulty. This jaw reconstruction can be achieved by extending the mandible with a rib graft or with the utilization of a distraction device.

The distraction of the mandible involves cutting the bones of the jaw (a corticotomy) and placing two pins on either side of the corticotomy. Each day, the pins are manually pushed apart and new bone is generated in the area of the corticotomy. The best approach to reconstructing the jaw is determined by the surgeon and is specific for each patient. If it is needed, ear reconstruction is performed in four stages and usually begins at the age of six years. Throughout life, these patients must maintain adequate dental occlusion through ongoing orthodontic treatment.

Information on this page is from: World Craniofacial Foundation, reprinted from their website at www.worldcf.org. © 1998; reprinted with permission.

Section 37.4

Treacher-Collins Syndrome

World Craniofacial Foundation, reprinted from their website at
www.worldcf.org. © 1998; reprinted with permission.

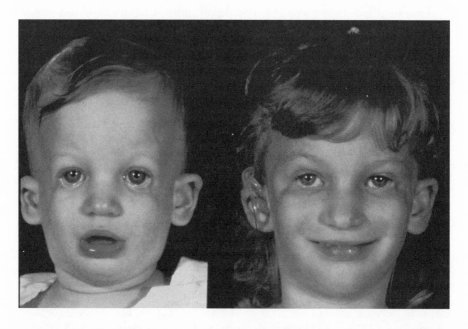

Figure 37.4. *Treacher-Collins Syndrome patient before and after surgery.*

Treacher-Collins Syndrome or Mandibulofacial Synostosis affects
the size and shape of the ears, cheek bones, and upper and lower jaws.
This condition is the result of an autosomal dominant gene.

Characteristics

The anomalies most often associated with this syndrome include:

- Facial cleft (Tessier 6-7-8 cleft),

- Hypoplasia of the cheeks and mandible bilaterally,

- Colobomas (or congenital scar) of the eyelids,

- Downward-sloping palpebral fissures,

- Poorly developed supraorbital rims and cheeks,

- Receding chin, and

- Malformation of the ear.

Although the severity of this syndrome can vary, the problems faced by a child with Treacher-Collins can be quite complicated and require the attention of a professional with experience with these types of patients. In the early years, patients often have difficulty maintaining an open airway and may need some assistance with obtaining adequate nutrition. In most cases as the patient grows and matures structurally, these problems are alleviated. Also, the malformation of the upper and lower jaws most often results in a malocclusion of the bite. A Treacher-Collins patient can also have impaired hearing depending upon the extent to which the deformity affects the formation of the ears. There may be a cleft of the palate as well.

Expectations

Children with Treacher-Collins Syndrome may have hypernasal resonance due to the presence of the cleft palate. Although most patients with this syndrome exhibit normal intelligence, some patients can have a decreased intellectual capacity. They may experience difficulty breathing and eating which they typically outgrow.

Treatment

Treacher-Collins patients generally require extensive care in the first few years of life. They may require the placement of a tracheostomy tube to assist them with breathing. A gastrostomy tube is used in the more severe cases to help the patient obtain adequate nutrition and energy for growth. Typically, these patients outgrow these problems and these tools are removed. Due to the severe underdevelopment of their upper and lower jaws, these patients usually require both mandibular and maxillary surgery to correct these deficits. The mandible can be corrected either by applying a rib graft to the mandible or through a technique known as distraction osteogenesis. The technique which will provide the best result will be decided on a cases by case basis by the craniofacial surgeon. With treatment of the jaws, it is necessary to obtain good orthodontic care to correct the malocclusion the deformity will produce. Nasal surgery may also be required to compensate for the deficient upper and lower jaws. In cases where colobomas exist, the children usually need eyelid reconstruction by a specialized pediatric ophthalmologist.

Section 37.5

Saethre-Chotzen Syndrome

World Craniofacial Foundation, reprinted from their website at
www.worldcf.org. © 1998; reprinted with permission.

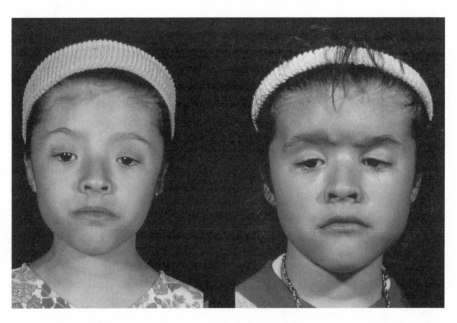

Figure 37.5. *Saethre-Chotzen Syndrome patient before and after surgery.*

Saethre-Chotzen Syndrome is a rare deformity that is closely related to Crouzon's Syndrome and both are thought to have similar
genetic origins.

Characteristics

Saethre-Chotzen Syndrome patients have some distinct features:

- Craniosynostosis most often of the coronal and lambdoid, and occasionally sagittal sutures,

- Underdeveloped mid-face which can be interpreted as either receded cheekbones or exophthalmus,

- Ocular Proptosis which is a prominence of the eyes due to very shallow orbits,

- Crossed eyes and/or wide-set eyes,

- Low set hairline, and

- Bilateral congenital ptosis or drooping of the upper eyelids.

Some other features commonly seen in these patients are visual disturbances related to an imbalance or absence of the muscle that moves the eyes, which usually requires surgery to correct. Also, ptosis of the eyelid is prevalent in these patients. There may be hearing loss due to recurrent ear infections. The mental capacity of these patients is usually in the normal range, however some mental delay has been reported.

Expectations

Children with Saethre-Chotzen Syndrome generally have normal intelligence although occasionally some reduced intellectual capacity can be seen. Because of the underdeveloped mid-face and high arched palate, nasal airway obstruction is not uncommon. Unusual resonance and speech patterns can develop from either the small nose, the high arched palate, or the malocclusion. A cleft palate can be associated with this syndrome and is repaired as it is with any other cleft patient. As with other cleft patients, there can be hearing problems due to recurrent ear infections. These patients may also experience difficulty with their vision. The presence of ptosis of the eyelids and the imbalance of absence of some of the muscles of the eye can contribute a great deal to this problem. Surgery is often required to correct this malformation. With proper treatment, these patients can be productive and active members of mainstream society.

Information on this page is from: World Craniofacial Foundation, reprinted from their website at www.worldcf.org. © 1998; reprinted with permission.

Treatment

Multiple-staged surgery is the general treatment plan for patients with Saethre-Chotzen Syndrome. In the first year of life it is preferred to release the synostotic sutures of the skull to allow adequate cranial volume to allow for brain growth and expansion. This procedure may need to be repeated in the life of the child. In addition, depending on the severity of the skull deformity, this procedure may be done in one stage or two stages. If necessary, mid-facial advancement and jaw surgery can be done to provide adequate orbital volume and reduce the exophthalmus and to correct the occlusion to an appropriate functional position. Eye muscle surgery often needs to be performed by a pediatric ophthalmologist to correct the imbalance in the muscular structures of the eye, as well as the ptosis of the eyelids.

Information on this page is from: World Craniofacial Foundation, reprinted from their website at www.worldcf.org. © 1998; reprinted with permission.

Section 37.6

Crouzon's Syndrome

World Craniofacial Foundation, reprinted from their website at
www.worldcf.org. © 1998; reprinted with permission.

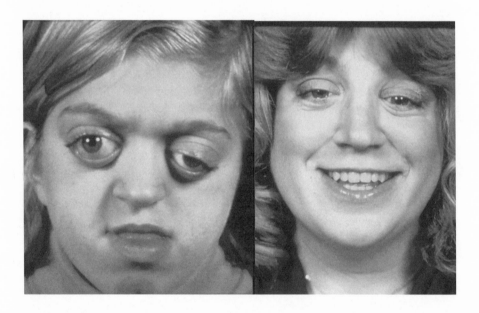

Figure 37.6. *Crouzon's patient before and after surgery.*

Crouzon's Syndrome, or craniofacial dystosis, is a rare deformity
that is closely related to Apert's Syndrome. Although many of the
physical deficiencies associated with Apert's are not present in the
Crouzon's patient, both are thought to have similar genetic origins.
Of the 10,000 infants born each day in the United States, it is estimated that one of these infants will have Crouzon's Syndrome.

Characteristics

Crouzon's Syndrome patients have these distinct features:

- Craniosynostosis most often of the coronal and lambdoid, and occasionally sagittal sutures,

- Underdeveloped mid-face with receded cheekbones or exophthalmos (bulging eyes),

- Ocular Proptosis which is a prominence of the eyes due to very shallow orbits, and

- Crossed eyes and/or wide-set eyes.

Some other features commonly seen in these patients are visual disturbances related to an imbalance of the muscle that move the eyes and hearing loss due to recurrent ear infections. The mental capacity of Crouzon's patients is usually in the normal range, however some mental delay has been reported.

Expectations

Children with Crouzon's Syndrome generally have normal intelligence although occasionally some reduced intellectual capacity can be seen. Because of the underdeveloped mid-face and high arched palate, nasal airway obstruction is not uncommon. Unusual resonance and speech patterns can develop from either the small nose, the high arched palate, or the malocclusion. A cleft palate can be associated with this syndrome and is repaired as it is with any other cleft patient. As with other cleft patients, there can be hearing problems due to recurrent ear infections. With proper treatment, these patients can be productive and active members of mainstream society.

Treatment

Multiple staged surgery is the general treatment plan for patients with Crouzon's Syndrome. In the first year of life it is preferred to release the synostotic sutures of the skull to allow adequate cranial volume to allow for brain growth and expansion. Skull reshaping may need to be repeated as the child grows to give the best possible

---

Information on this page is from: World Craniofacial Foundation, reprinted from their website at www.worldcf.org. © 1998; reprinted with permission.

191

results. In addition, depending on the severity of the skull deformity, this procedure may be done in one stage or two stages. If necessary, mid-facial advancement and jaw surgery can be done to provide adequate orbital volume and reduce the exophthalmus to correct the occlusion to an appropriate functional position and to provide for a more normal appearance.

Information on this page is from: World Craniofacial Foundation, reprinted from their website at www.worldcf.org. © 1998; reprinted with permission.

Section 37.7

Carpenter's Syndrome

World Craniofacial Foundation, reprinted from their website at
www.worldcf.org. © 1998; reprinted with permission.

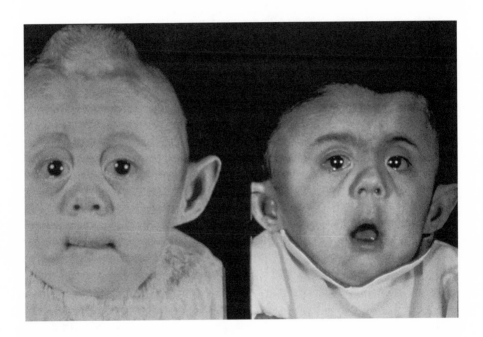

Figure 37.7. *Carpenter's Syndrome patient before and after surgery.*

Carpenter's Syndrome is a very rare craniofacial condition. There
are approximately 40 reported cases to date and it occurs as an autosomal recessive inherited gene.

Characteristics

The physical manifestation of Carpenter's Syndrome is character-ized by and include:

- Tower shaped skull,
- Presence of additional or fused fingers and toes,
- Reduced height,
- Obesity, and
- Mental deficiency.

Often associated with this defect is marked cranial asymmetry described as a "cloverleaf" skull anomaly caused by the craniosynos-tosis. Also, there is mild down sloping of the eyes, epicanthal folds, as well as malformations of the eyes themselves. The ears of these patients are low set, their necks are short, and their mandible may be somewhat small. Commonly seen in these patients is a highly arched and somewhat narrow palate. The mental deficiency seen with these patients varies from mild to severe, although multiple cases have been reported with normal intelligence.

Expectations

Patients with Carpenter's Syndrome can have some problems with speech due to the presence of the highly arched and vaulted palate. The growth of these patients is limited by the syndrome. They usu-ally exhibit a short, stock stature.

Treatment

Due to the extremely low frequency of these cases, the treatment plans vary greatly from patient to patient. The treatment plan usually includes surgery in the first year of life to correct their cranial deformity. This is performed first to insure there is adequate volume of the cranial vault to support the rapid growth of the brain during this period of life. These procedures may need to be done in one stage or two stages depending on the degree of the deformity. If necessary, mid-face advancement and jaw surgery are done to provide adequate orbital volume and appropri-ate occlusion. Hand reconstruction is done early in life by a plastic sur-geon hand specialist to allow for the best functional results.

Information on this page is from: World Craniofacial Foundation, reprinted from their website at www.worldcf.org. © 1998; reprinted with permission.

Section 37.8

Apert's Syndrome

World Craniofacial Foundation, reprinted from their website at www.worldcf.org. © 1998; reprinted with permission.

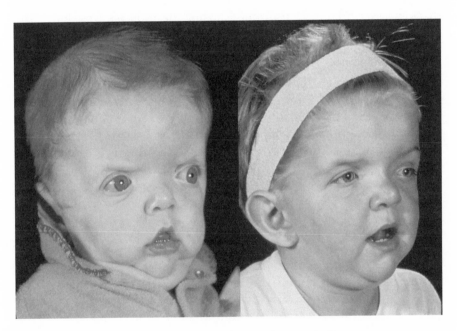

Figure 37.8. *Apert's Syndrome patient before and after surgery.*

Apert's Syndrome is a relatively uncommon craniofacial condition. It occurs with a frequency of one in 160,000 live births. The condition may be inherited with a frequency of 50% in the off-spring of an affected adult, or may develop as a spontaneous mutation.

Characteristics

The physical features of this condition were described by Frederick Apert in 1942 and include:

- A tower-shaped skull due to craniosynostosis,

- An under-developed mid-face leading to recessed cheek bones and prominent eyes,

- Malocclusion, and

- Limb abnormalities such as webbing of the middle digits of the hands and feet.

Some other features commonly seen in this condition are visual disturbances related to an imbalance of the muscles that move the eyes, a hearing loss due to recurrent ear infections, and varying degrees of acne. There can be a reduced intellectual capacity in some individuals but there are some children with this condition who have normal intelligence. Children with Apert's have fusion of the bones of their fingers and toes, characterized by the "mitten-like" appearance of their hands. This is called syndactyly. Cardiac and gastrointestinal malformations may be present in Apert's patients which have not been described for those individuals with other syndromes.

Expectations

Children with Apert's Syndrome may have unusual speech characteristics. They often have hyponasal resonance due to an under-developed mid-face, small nose, and excessively long soft palate. If there is a cleft palate, they may also have hypernasal resonance. Articulation of speech sounds is often distorted due to the malocclusion and high arched palate. Impaired hearing or a general developmental delay will also effect speech and language development.

Treatment

Multiple staged surgery is the plan of treatment for children with Apert's. The best time for release of the fused sutures is between three and six months of age; it may be performed up to 18 months of age.

Information on this page is from: World Craniofacial Foundation, reprinted from their website at www.worldcf.org. © 1998; reprinted with permission.

This early surgery allows the child's brain to have plenty of room to grow. Besides release of other sutures, the frontal and other deformed bones will be repositioned (usually advanced) to correct the bulging eyes and upper facial deformities. The plastic surgeon and the neurosurgeon work with one another in the operating room to achieve the end result. If the mid-face and upper jaw still do not grow adequately, this procedure may need to be repeated in adolescence. The webbing of the fingers is normally addressed by separation of the digits in the first years of life in order to achieve better alignment and function of the hand. Sometimes, this may require several procedures to give the child adequate function.

Information on this page is from: World Craniofacial Foundation, reprinted from their website at www.worldcf.org. © 1998; reprinted with permission.

Section 37.9

Pfeiffer's Syndrome

World Craniofacial Foundation, reprinted from their website at
www.worldcf.org. © 1998; reprinted with permission.

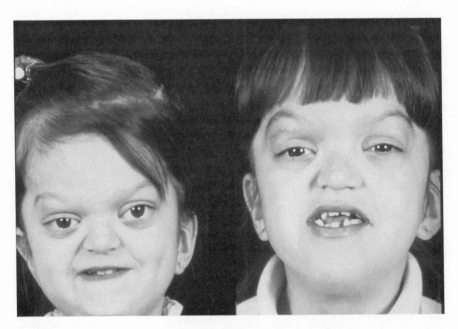

Figure 37.9. *Pfeiffer's Syndrome patient before and after surgery.*

Pfeiffer's Syndrome, like the other craniosynostotic Syndromes, is
caused by a genetic mutation. The physical manifestations of this
Syndrome match those of Crouzon's and include broad thumbs and
toes.

Characteristics

Pfeiffer's Syndrome patients have the following abnormalities:

- Craniosynostosis most often of the coronal and lambdoid, and occasionally sagittal sutures,

- Underdeveloped mid-face with receded cheekbones or exophthalmos,

- Ocular Proptosis which is a prominence of the eyes due to very shallow orbits,

- Crossed eyes and/or wide-set eyes, and

- Broad thumbs and big toes.

Some other features commonly seen in these patients are visual disturbances related to an imbalance of the muscle that move the eyes and hearing loss due to recurrent ear infections. The mental capacity of Pfeiffer patients is usually in the normal range, however some mental delay has been reported.

Expectations

Children with Pfeiffer's Syndrome generally have normal intelligence although occasionally some reduced intellectual capacity can be seen. Because of the underdeveloped mid-face and high arched palate, nasal airway obstruction is not uncommon. Unusual resonance and speech patterns can develop from either the small nose, the high arched palate, or the malocclusion. A cleft palate can be associated with this syndrome and is repaired as it is with any other cleft patient. As with other cleft patients, there can be hearing problems due to recurrent ear infections. With proper treatment, these patients can be productive and active members of mainstream society.

Treatment

Multiple staged surgery is the general treatment plan for patients with Pfeiffer's Syndrome. In the first year of life it is preferred to release the synostotic sutures of the skull to allow adequate cranial volume to allow for brain growth and expansion. Skull remodeling

---

Information on this page is from: World Craniofacial Foundation, reprinted from their website at www.worldcf.org. © 1998; reprinted with permission.

may need to be repeated as the child grows. If necessary, mid-facial advancement and jaw surgery can be done to provide adequate orbital volume and reduce the exophthalmos and to correct the occlusion to an appropriate functional position. Although there is a significant malformation of the fingers and toes, usually these function adequately and do not require the surgical attention of a plastic surgeon hand specialist.

Information on this page is from: World Craniofacial Foundation, reprinted from their website at www.worldcf.org. © 1998; reprinted with permission.

Chapter 38

Congenital Anomalies of the Hand

Summary

This manuscript reviews the basic and most common types of congenital hand anomalies seen by the pediatrician. Each disorder is categorized into the standard classification system used, and the main highlights of each condition are detailed with representative illustrations. Other system anomalies associated with congenital hand problems are also identified.

Introduction

Nary a new mother will pass 24 hours without counting the number of fingers and toes on her newborn. Congenital hand anomalies are noted very quickly after birth and can cause parents some consternation with what otherwise may have been a happy and uncomplicated event. Furthermore, congenital deformities of the hand account for approximately 6% to 7% of all admissions to children's hospital services in the United States.

Classification of congenital hand anomalies has been a difficult task, with more than 50 classification systems drafted over the past 150 years. Currently, hand surgeons use the system adopted by both

"Congenital Anomalies of the Hand," by Jonathan G. Smith, MMS, Arnold-Peter C. Weiss, MD, and Yvonne S. Weiss, MD., *Clinical Pediatrics*, August 1998, vol. 3, pp.459-468. © 1998 Westminster Publications, Inc.; reprinted with permission.

the American Society for Surgery of the Hand and the International Federation of Societies for Surgery of the Hand. A summary of this system, first presented by Swanson, is provided here as Table 38.1. The following review aims to provide a concise summary of some of the more common congenital anomalies of the hand encountered in pediatric medicine and is based on the aforementioned classification system.

Table 38.1. Summary of Swanson Classification System for Congenital Hand Anomalies

I.   Failure of formation of parts (arrest of development)

         Transverse deficiencies: amputation-arm, forearm, wrist, hand, digits

         Longitudinal deficiencies: radial club hand, ulnar club hand, cleft hand

II.   Failure of differentiation (separation) of parts

         Symphalangism

         Camptodactyly

         Clinodactyly

         Trigger thumb

         Syndactyly: simple, complex, part of associated syndrome

III.   Duplication

         Polydactyly

         Triphalangeal thumb

IV.   Overgrowth

         Macrodactyly

V.   Undergrowth

         Thumb Hypoplasia

VI.   Congenital constriction band syndrome

VII.   Generalized skeletal abnormalities

I. Failure of Formation of Parts

Transverse Deficiencies

Transverse or terminal failures of formation are those in which there are no normal parts distal to the point of the anomaly. Congenital amputations, complete absence of a body part, may be encountered at any level of the upper extremity, ranging from amelia (absence of the entire limb) to aphalangia (absence of the phalanges). Muscular deficiencies are often seen with these conditions. The most frequently occurring defect in this class is the below-elbow (BE) amputation, frequently attributable to thalidomide. BE amputations are seen most commonly in females on the left side.

While the new parents are bound to be alarmed by these anomalies, they may be somewhat relieved to learn that surgery is seldom necessary in these cases.-. rather, prosthetics are usually the preferred method of treatment and often provide excellent functional status. The infant may begin to be fit for a prosthesis as early as 3 months of age, with revision prostheses as the child ages. Other treatment options may include ablation, lengthening, and microvascular transfer, or, of course, keeping the status quo. With appropriate treatment, the prognosis for these children is excellent functionally.

Longitudinal Deficiencies

Longitudinal deficiencies are defined as those involving a "unique arrest of formation identified by using the absent bone's name." Radial club hand, simply defined, is a congenital absence of the radius. The defect is reported to have an incidence of 1:100,000 and may be unilateral, or bilateral. Presentation occurs at birth as either a partial or total absence of the radial side of the forearm and hand, causing radial deviation of the affected wrist(s), and a fixed flexion contracture of the elbow(s). Additionally, the ulna appears shortened and curved on radiographs (Figures 38.1. A, B). As with many of the congenital anomalies, numerous structures may be affected. For example, hypoplasia of the thumb, with accompanying absence of the first metacarpal, may or may not be present. Severe cases are more likely to involve not only the thumb but also other structures along the radial aspect of the forearm, such as the radial artery and nerve, and adjacent tendons. In addition, one may note absence or fusion of the carpal bones. While numerous combinations are possible, the most common pattern consists of partial absence of the radius, carpus, and thumb.

The physician, often the pediatrician, who first discovers one of these anomalies in a child should pay particular heed to these radial defects, for they quite often prove to be part of a larger associated disorder: 77% of cases "I show involvement of other organ systems, 95% when the radial deficiency is bilateral. Cardiac (most commonly septal defects explained by the fact that the cardiac septum forms at the same time as the radius) or gastrointestinal (GI) (most commonly imperforate anus) anomalies are frequent in these patients, and prompt attention with a thorough physical examination is therefore critical. In addition, thrombocytopenia-absent radius (TAR) syndrome (usually present at birth with severe deficiency of platelets, which generally resolves in 12 to 18 months) should be ruled out, particularly in patients who present with a bilateral radial club hand. The VATER association, Holt-Oram syndrome, and Fanconi's anemia are other conditions associated with radial club deformity. Possible genitourinary abnormalities should likewise be evaluated by means of ultrasonography or an intravenous pyelogram to rule out unilateral renal agenesis.

Initial treatment consists of serial casting and/or manipulation with passive stretching techniques. If the elbow is of normal character

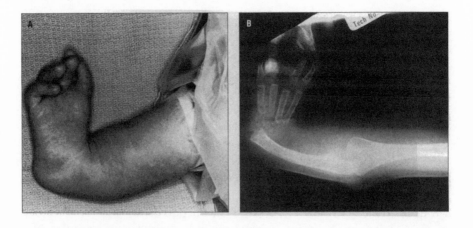

Figure 38.1. A, B Young boy has normal elbow function with a radial club hand and complete absence of the thumb (A). Note the "pollicizing attitude" of the index finger, which frequently begins acting as the thumb would. Radiographs (B) demonstrate complete absence of the radius.

and passive correction can be achieved, patients are treated surgically. Surgical correction, typically performed at 6 to 12 months of age, aims to stabilize the hand on the forearm via a centralization procedure of the wrist on the distal ulna. This procedure was first described in 1893 and has been modified and revised repeatedly, leading to "radialization," described nearly 100 years later. The ulna may be severely curved and may require multiple osteotomies with a central pin fixation in order to try to improve both length and cosmetic appearance. Patients with a hypoplastic or absent thumb typically require pollicization of the index finger for functional pinch.

Pollicization is a procedure whereby the index finger is shortened and transferred into the thumb position surgically. Occasionally, children are seen in whom the index finger undertakes a migration to a "pollicized" state. In such a case, formal surgical pollicization may not be indicated or required.

Congenital absence of the ulna is another longitudinal deficiency seen far less commonly than radial anomalies. In contrast to radial club hand, ulnar club patients exhibit defects at the elbow, with a stable wrist. In addition, the cardiac and GI conditions commonly associated with radial club hand are usually not present in ulnar club cases. As with the radial defects, however, surgical correction is usually indicated at an early age in order to create a one-bone forearm.

Cleft hand, or central hypoplasia of the hand, is the other major type of congenital anomaly found in this first class of the Swanson classification system. This condition usually carries autosomal dominant inheritance and is often bilateral. Longitudinal absence of the central ray of the hand gives the hand an appearance of a lobster claw, giving the anomaly its unfortunate slang term "lobster claw hand." Seemingly absent fingers may in fact be aplastic or may be fused to adjacent digits, causing the claw appearance (Figure 38.2.). This has been termed ectrodactyly and often creates hands (usually bilateral) that have satisfactory functional capacity but undesirable appearance. Surgical repair for this condition involves early closure of the cleft and subsequent reconstruction between the index and ring fingers. As with other defects of this class, functional prognosis following surgery is usually good.

II. Failure of Differentiation (Separation) of Parts

The second class of congenital hand anomalies accounts for many of the more frequently encountered defects. In contrast to the first class in which structures fail to form, anomalies seen here involve structures that form incorrectly.

Symphalangism is an autosomal dominant condition involving stiffness in the proximal interphalangeal (PIP) joints of the fingers. The anomaly is often present bilaterally and is most likely to affect the little finger. Stiffness is due to fusion of the proximal and middle phalanges, resulting in locked extension of the affected digit(s). Imaging may reveal bony ankylosis or severely altered joint surfaces with minimal joint space. This condition is generally not treated. Arthroplasty of the affected digit(s) remains an option, yet good functional status is usually seen in these children, often precluding the necessity for surgery.

Camptodactyly is another autosomal dominant failure of differentiation. Unlike some of the other anomalies, however, camptodactyly is not usually seen in the neonate (although neonatal cases are possible).

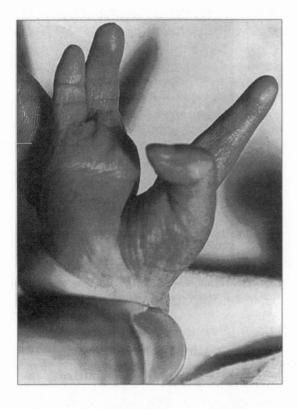

Figure 38.2. A young girl demonstrates a significant cleft hand with absence of the middle finger and its assorted metacarpal.

On the contrary, variations of the condition may present in infancy or in early adolescence. Patients present with a congenital flexion deformity usually at the PIP joint, most commonly affecting the little finger (Figure 38.3.). The etiology behind the soft tissue contracture causing the flexion deformity is poorly understood, although it generally relates to an abnormal insertion of the lumbrical muscles or the flexor digitorum superficialis tendon.

Treatment for these cases relies largely on splinting. While serial splinting is recommended as the primary treatment, outcome has been variable. Another option to consider for treating these cases is surgical release of the contracture, yet this type of procedure is technically demanding and frequently yields less than optimal results. With flexion contractures of greater than 60 degrees, operative intervention may prove useful.

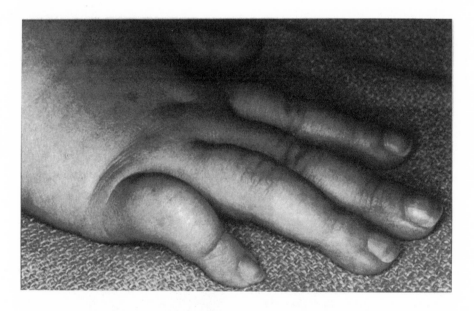

Figure 38.3. *A girl presents with congenital bending of the proximal interphalangeal (PIP) joint of the small finger—camptodactyly.*

Clinodactyly refers to a curvature of the digit in the coronal (or radioulnar) plane. It is most commonly seen in the small finger and next frequently in the thumb (Figure 38.4.). The deformity is usually noted at the distal interphalangeal (DIP) joint, with the distal portion of the finger tilting toward the midline of the hand. This generally involves abnormal growth of the distal aspect of the involved phalanx, but in severe cases can also involve an extra bone termed the "delta phalanx." The condition frequently carries a family history and is also commonly bilateral. Unless significant scissoring of the digits occurs, treatment is generally undertaken for cosmetic reasons only. A closing or opening wedge osteotomv can be performed with excellent functional results.

Trigger thumb, or stenosing tenovaginitis of the thumb. is a fixed flexion contracture of the interphalangeal joint. The condition may be recognized at birth, but in most cases it is first noticed in young children (adults may also suffer from trigger thumb or finger, but in

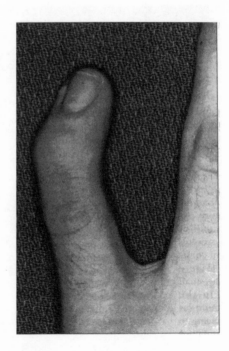

Figure 38.4. A teenage boy with clinodactyly—radial deviation of the distal interphalangeal (DIP) joint. He notes no inhibition of function.

these cases the condition is acquired, not congenital). The deformity is frequently overlooked at first owing to the neonate's clenching of the fist. It can go unnoticed for an extended period of time by the parents, yet once noticed, it causes substantial distress. A palpable nodule observable at the metacarpal head is a localized swelling of the flexor pollicis longus (FPL) tendon, which prevents the FPL tendon from completing its normal excursion, thereby preventing active extension of the joint. Passive extension is also painful in many of these patients. The condition involves the thumb far more frequently than any other digit and in some cases will resolve without surgical treatment. Thus, initial treatment should be conservative, with splinting and/or stretching as needed. Spontaneous resolution has been reported in 30% of cases found at birth. If the condition does not resolve itself, however, then surgical release of the A-1 pulley at the metacarpal head is recommended. This usually provides immediate relief, and patients usually recover full function soon after surgery. One must be cautious not to wait too long to operate, however, for it has been noted that residual flexion contracture has been observed in patients older than 4 years of age at the time of surgery.

Syndactyly refers to a fusion of adjacent digits due to intrauterine failure to separate. This phenotype may present as either a 'simple' syndactyly in which all phalangeal joints are normal and the fusion involves only the skin and soft tissue, or it may present as 'complex' syndactyly in which there is bony union. The distinction between simple and complex can be made by means of plain radiographs. Furthermore, the condition is considered 'complete' if the soft tissue between the digits is united as far as the distal phalanx, or 'incomplete' if it is united short of the distal phalanx. Unlike many of the congenital anomalies, syndactyly may be easily diagnosed at birth. The condition may be either unilateral or bilateral and is most frequently seen between the middle and ring fingers. Webbing between the ring and little fingers is the second most common type, comprising 25% of cases. The thumb may be involved, although these cases are least frequent.

Syndactyly is the most common congenital anomaly in Caucasians and often presents with a positive family history when the condition presents alone. In addition, syndactyly is frequently seen as a characteristic of more generalized disorders such as Poland's and Apert's syndromes. Poland's syndrome involves hypoplasia of the entire extremity with bradysyndactyly, or syndactyly with short fingers of the ipsilateral hand. Apert's syndrome involves complete syndactyly of all fingers, with a spoon-shaped palm and common fingernail (Figure 38.5).

Surgical release is indicated in order to improve both function and appearance and is generally performed at 6 months of age. The procedure should be performed no later than 3 to 4 years of age in order to provide normal development of movement and dexterity. Cases involving syndactyly between digits of unequal length should be released at an early age in order to prevent any secondary deformity due to asymmetric growth of the fingers. In addition, early release is indicated in complex cases involving bony union at the distal aspects of the fingers. Release should not be performed simultaneously on adjacent webs on both sides of one digit, however, since this may give rise to excessive skin loss. Prognosis is highly variable and is particularly dependent on the presence or absence of associated conditions described above. In syndactyly cases involving the toes, surgical correction is often not required, since functional capacity is not usually impaired.

III. Duplication

Failures of formation and differentiation are two of the three most common congenital hand anomalies. Duplication defects complete this trio.

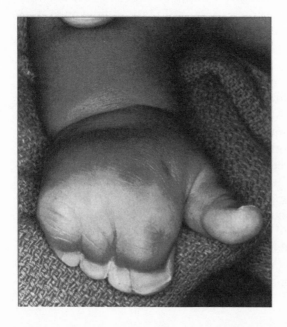

Figure 38.5. A young child with Apert's syndrome demonstrates the most severe form of syndactyly with all fingers fused forming a "mitten hand" and with some fusing of the nailbeds.

Polydactyly, or supernumerary digits, rivals syndactyly as the most common congenital anomaly. This condition is more frequently seen in the thumb or small finger and usually presents with more phalanges than corresponding metacarpals (Figures 38. 6A, B). Duplication of the small finger is often seen in the African-American population (as frequently as 1 in 100) owing to an autosomal dominant trait and usually presents as an isolated finding. This same anomaly is seen in Caucasian children much less commonly and, when present, is frequently associated with other anomalies such as Ellis von Crevald syndrome, requiring a complete and thorough physical examination. In many cases, patients will be affected bilaterally, with possible involvement of the toes. While the extra digit is seen both grossly and with radiologic imaging, the patient usually does not have voluntary control over it.

Duplication in its simplest form involves a small piece of extra soft tissue without bony elements that can be tied off in the nursery without resulting cosmetic deformity. This type of polydactyly is encountered more frequently than it is actually reported, which may in fact make polydactyly the most common congenital anomaly.

Larger duplications involving soft tissue and/or bone require surgical removal. Some complicated forms of duplication in the thumb

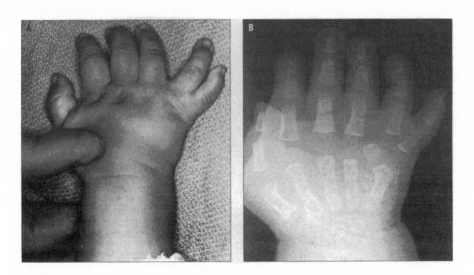

Figure 38.6. A, B *An otherwise healthy boy has duplication of the small finger (A), and radiographs (B) reveal a complex partial duplication of the metacarpal heads.*

211

or in the central digits become difficult reconstructive procedures owing to the requirement of maintaining a functionally stable joint after the reconstruction. Such reconstructions may not only involve removal but may also entail combination and/or revision procedures. Nevertheless, surgical correction for this condition is quite successful with ideal timing at 1 year of age.

Triphalangeal thumb is another, less common, congenital anomaly due to duplication and is frequently familial. This may occur with thumb polydactyly, as part of the Holt-Oran syndrome, or it may present as a solitary condition. The duplication in these cases presents as an extra phalanx between the two normal phalanges of the thumb. The defect may present as three normal size phalanges, giving the thumb a long appearance; a finger-like thumb, giving rise to the 'five-fingered hand'; or a small wedge-shaped delta phalanx, causing the thumb to bend toward the index finger.

Surgical treatment for triphalangeal thumb is usually recommended. One of the phalanges is removed, and the thumb is shortened to normal length. If webbing of the thumb needs to be released, this is done as well. In cases involving a delta phalanx, the bone should either be removed prior to age 1 year or fused to one of the normal phalanges in an older child (Figure 38.7). Additionally, in the case of the five-fingered hand, a pollicization procedure is performed in order to provide opposition function of the thumb. Functional prognosis following surgery is usually good.

IV. Overgrowth

As mentioned previously, the majority of congenital hand anomalies fall into the three categories discussed above. In this section and the ones to follow, a brief description of defects seen in remaining classes is offered. Macrodactyly is a rare congenital anomaly in which there is excessive growth of a digit. Hypertrophy, may result from developmental anomalies or may be a manifestation of neurofibromatosis. A complete evaluation is therefore necessary in order to rule out a greater underlying etiology. Two main types of macrodactyly may be seen: the static type of macrodactyly presents as an enlarged digit at birth, and the affected finger grows proportionally as the child grows. In contrast, the affected digit in patients with a disproportionate-type anomaly grows faster than other fingers. This may be due to excessive stimulation of nerves and is likely to affect multiple adjacent digits.

The wide variety of possible phenotypes within this family of anomalies is matched by a corresponding gamut of treatment options.

In the case of the neonate, no treatment is indicated. In cases where treatment is attempted, earlier treatment is more likely to succeed, although no surgical procedure is known to have a predictably favorable outcome. Removal of fat, epiphyseal arrest of involved phalanges, and complete ablation have been cited as possible strategies for surgical correction. Given the spectrum of possible presentations and limited surgical options, however, prognosis is highly variable and not terribly favorable in many cases.

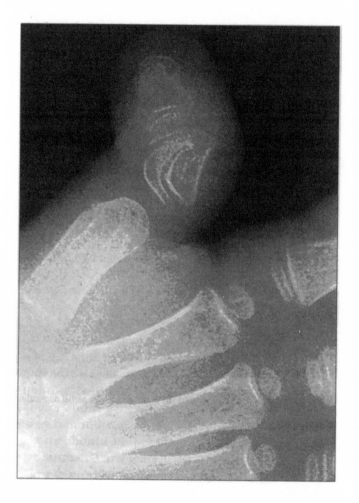

Figure 38.7. *Radiographs of a child with severe radial deviation of the thumb demonstrate a delta phalanx with its "C" shaped epiphysis.*

V. Undergrowth

In addition to cases involving overgrowth of parts of the hand, another class of defects involves undergrowth or hypoplasias of the hand. Thumb hypoplasia is one of the more common examples of undergrowth. Complete absence of the thumb may be considered to be a failure of formation or may be considered the most severe form of thumb hypoplasia. Congenital thumb hypoplasia is defined as failing to extend to the level of the PIP joint of the index finger.

Treatment for hypoplasia cases is once again dependant on the specific presentation of the individual case. In most cases, functional loss is minimal, and therefore surgery may not be necessary. In other cases, however, surgical lengthening of the thumb may be indicated, sometimes requiring surgical transfer of the first or second toe to the thumb. In cases involving complete absence of the thumb, pollicization of the index finger is indicated, as discussed above in section I. Prognosis for undergrowth cases is often quite good given the appropriate surgical corrections.

VI. Congenital Constriction Band Syndrome

The etiology of constriction band syndrome is not clear, but commonly, associated signs and anomalies are seen in the extremities, particularly the fingers and toes. Such anomalies may include various combinations of defects described above. Amputations may be found, owing to distal necrosis in utero. Cases in which the band is not tight enough to induce necrosis may result in edema, leading to hypoplastic digits. Additionally, in cases involving a superficial constriction, one may find varying degrees of syndactyly.

Surgical release of the band is urgent if and only if the child is born with edema with a viable digit. Necrotic digits are not candidates for repair by surgical release, for the damage is irreversible. Children presenting with superficial syndactyly should be treated surgically by use of Z-plasty procedures at six months of age, with later surgical reconstructions as needed. Prognosis is highly variable from case to case.

VII. Generalized Skeletal Abnormalities

This category of congenital hand problems is quite broad and beyond the scope of this limited discussion. Many of the conditions seen in this category are chromosomal in nature and lead to specific anatomical variations. Madelung's deformity is one such disorder which involves abnormal growth on the ulnar half of the distal radius. It is more common in females and most often bilateral, and its appearance becomes more prevalent in adolescence. Limited wrist range of motion is generally present, and the cosmetic deformity is relatively mild although present. The diagnosis can be made on radiographic examination, and treatment is only rendered if the condition becomes significantly symptomatic, which is generally uncommon.

Discussion

The major hand anomalies can be successfully treated from a functional perspective, although in the vast majority of children some cosmetic deformity still remains. A large body of extremely rare or unusual congenital conditions also exist that require more complex evaluation and treatment and are beyond the scope of this review.

In evaluating the newborn, the physician should pay very close heed to suspected or obvious anomalies of the hand. As noted above, many of these anomalies are frequently part of a larger syndrome or sequence, and any suspicion of such a condition should be worked up completely. Associated cardiac or GI anomalies must be ruled out or diagnosed so that they can be addressed before leading to greater problems for the child and the new parents.

In addition, assigning a classification or diagnosis may sometimes prove difficult. In many cases as described above, the child may present with combinations of anomalies, as in cases of radial club hand. In these cases, the physician frequently encounters difficulty in discerning the causal relationship among existing deficiencies and must try to diagnose the underlying etiology. In addition, one may encounter cases involving radiology of bone that has not yet ossified. In such cases, the best option may be to withhold treatment until a later date when a definitive diagnosis can be made with greater confidence. Multiple factors such as the maturity of the bone, joints, and nervous system of the patient, as well as the patient's developmental stage and anesthetic risk, are key factors in deciding when to perform a surgical procedure. The physician should keep close watch over these patients and work closely with the parents so that they understand that their child may have a potential problem even though it might not be possible to label it with an absolute diagnosis at birth.

Children with congenital hand anomalies frequently require multiple procedures over a prolonged period of time. Fortunately, in many cases various means of treatment and/or therapy are available, and there are few things more rewarding than establishing a relationship with these children and their parents.

Chapter 39

Skin Grafts for Burns

A first degree or superficial burn heals naturally through the body's ability to replace damaged skin cells. Deep second and full thickness burns require skin graft surgery for quick healing and minimal scarring. In the case of large burn size, patients will need more than one operation during a hospital stay.

Patients may need surgery for surgical debridment (cleaning). Skin grafting is also done in surgery, which consists of excision or the surgical removal of burn injured tissue; choosing a donor site, or an area from which healthy skin is removed to be used as cover for the cleaned burned area; and harvesting, where the graft is removed from the donor site by an instrument similar to an electric shaver. This instrument (dermatome) gently shaves a piece of skin, about 10/1000 of an inch thick, off the unburned area. Finally, the surgeon places and secures the skin graft over the surgically cleaned wound so that it can heal.

Skin donated by other people who have died (called homograft, allograft, or cadaver skin) is sometimes used as a temporary cover for a burned area that has been cleaned. To help the graft heal and become secure, the area of the graft is not moved for five days following each surgery (immobilization period). During this immobilization period, blood vessels begin to grow from the tissue below into the donor skin, bonding the two layers together. Five days after grafting, exercise therapy programs, tub baths and other normal daily activities resume.

In smaller burns, where the sheet-like cover of the epidermis is burned away, the resulting wound heals by lateral overgrowth of the epithelial cells living in the skin appendages (healing occurs as the edges of the wound grow until they cover the area). A wound two centimeters in diameter will heal in about ten days. Most deep partial-thickness burns and third-degree burns larger than three centimeters in diameter are best treated with early excision (removal of dead tissue), immediate skin grafting, and long-term use of compression garments to minimize hypertrophic scarring.

When a wound is larger than two centimeters, or if the edges can't pull themselves together (for example over the heel or knee, where there is tension with each movement), the wound becomes a chronic ulcer (open area) and never closes. A skin graft is a better solution for this type of wound.

Skin graft surgery is recommended for burns that are deep. All skin grafting is done in surgery where patients can be anesthetized before the procedure. A skin graft surgery is done to replace skin that is lost

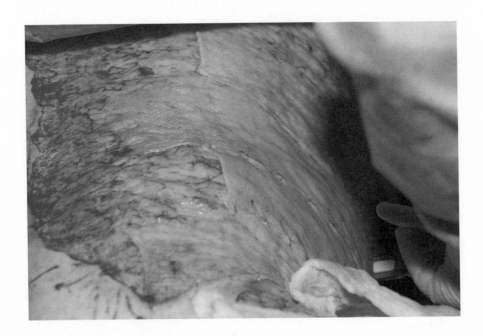

Figure 39.1. Skin Graft Surgery

or has been damaged. During the skin graft surgery, the dead burned skin is cut away. This cutting away and cleaning down to healthy tissue is called excision. The second part of a skin graft surgery is to repair the excised burn area by covering it with donor skin. Donor skin is a patch of healthy skin that is transplanted, or moved, from another area of the body. A skin graft, where the donor skin is taken from some other part of the burn-injured person, is called an autograft (from oneself). Family members often ask if they can donate (give) their skin for the graft operation. The answer is "No." Permanent donor skin has to come from the person who was burned, or the skin will be rejected and it will slough and will not heal the wound.

Doctors who do operations are called surgeons. They work in bright, airy operating rooms (surgery rooms) where everything is very clean. All of the tools used in surgery are sterile—free from germs or dirt! To keep germs away from the patients, surgeons and nurses also wear caps, face masks, rubber gloves, and gowns.

During surgery an anesthetic is used. An anesthetic is a substance that produces loss of feeling. A general anesthetic does this by making the patient unconscious. Some anesthetics are given by injection into a vein (intravenous injection) and others are given as a gas mixture, which is breathed into the lungs and then absorbed into the bloodstream.

Often burn patients need blood transfusions to replace blood lost during surgery. Blood transfusions increase the red blood cells, which carry oxygen from the lungs to every part of the body and take waste carbon dioxide back to the lungs, where it is breathed out into the air. If there aren't enough red blood cells or if the cells do not contain enough iron to carry oxygen properly, wounds do not heal as well.

Temporary Wound Covering

Allograft, cadaver skin, or homograft is human cadaver skin donated for medical use. The clinical use of allograft skin in the modern era was popularized by James Barrett Brown, who described its use in 1942. Cadaver skin is used as a temporary covering for excised (cleaned) wound surfaces before autograft (permanent) placement. Unmeshed cadaver is put over the excised wound and stapled in place. Post-operatively, the cadaver may be covered with a dressing. Wound coverage using cadaveric allograft is removed prior to permanent autografting. Xenograft or heterograft is skin taken from a variety of animals, usually a pig. Heterograft skin became popular because of the limited availability and high expense of human skin tissue. In some cases religious, financial, or cultural objections to the use of human cadaver skin may also be factors. Wound coverage using xenograft or heterograft is a temporary covering used until autograft. Porcine is commonly used as temporary skin coverage for Exfoliative Skin Diseases (e.g., SJS, TEN).

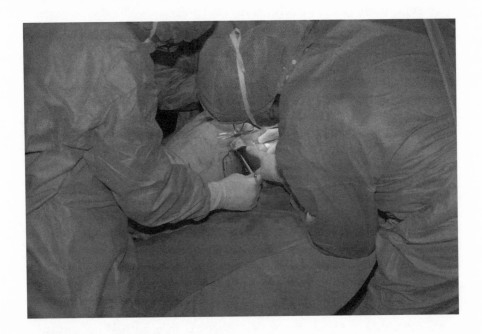

Figure 39.2. *A staple skin graft.*

Permanent Wound Covering

An **autograft** is skin taken from the person burned, which is used to cover wounds permanently. Since the skin is a major organ in the body, an autograft is essentially an organ transplant. Autograft is surgically removed using a dermatome (a tool with a sharp razor blade). A dermatome sheers the donor skin off the body. Only the top layer of skin is used for donor skin. Donor skin is taken at such a depth where the site will heal on its own, very similar to a second degree burn. There are two types of autografts used for permanent wound coverage: sheet grafts and meshed grafts.

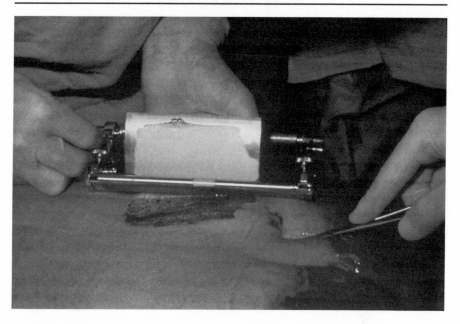

Figure 39.3. Surgeons use a dermatome to remove skin.

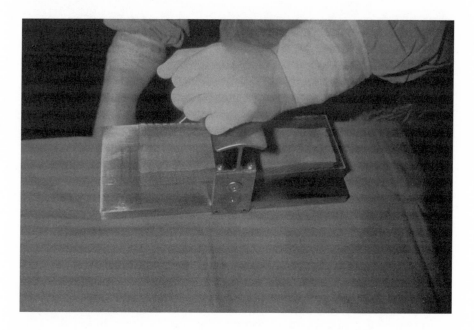

Figure 39.4. Surgeons use a mesher to put holes in grafted skin.

How the Doctors Get Donor Skin

A dermatome (a tool with a sharp razor blade) sheers the donor skin off the body. Only the top layer of skin is used for donor skin. Donor skin thickness is usually .010 to .014 inches thick.

Types of Skin Grafts

Sheet Grafts

For a sheet graft, a piece of donor skin is removed from an un-burned area of the body. The size of the donor skin that is used to patch a burned area is about the same size. No slits or holes are put into a sheet graft. Because the donor skin used in sheet grafts is not stretched, it takes a larger donor site to cover the same area. When a burn is large, sheet grafts are saved for the face, neck and hands—

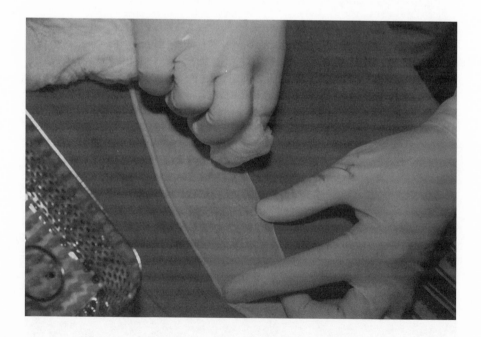

Figure 39.5. A sheet graft is skin removed from an unburned part of the body.

making the most visible parts of the body appear less scarred. When a burn is small, and there is plenty of donor skin to use, a sheet graft is usually used to cover the burned area. A disadvantage of a sheet graft is that there is a possibility for small areas of graft loss from build up of fluid under the sheet right after surgery. Sheet graft is usually more durable and it leaves fewer scars so it is less noticeable.

Meshed Skin Grafts

Very large areas of open wounds, such as a major burn, are difficult to cover because there might not be enough unburned door skin available. Skin grafts that are placed as a sheet look better after they heal, but require an area of donor skin as big as the burned area. For covering larger areas, donor skin can be meshed.

In a meshed skin graft, the skin from the donor site is stretched to allow it to cover an area larger than itself. This involves making

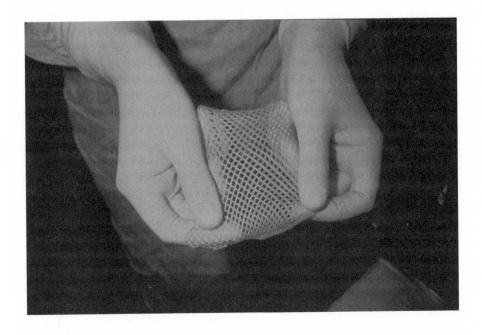

Figure 39.6. *A mesh graft is skin that has small slits put in it, allowing it to expand like a fish net.*

small slits in the skin which allow it to expand like fish netting. The spaces between the slits in the donor skin heal by growing back together. The disadvantages of meshing are 1) it is a less durable graft than a sheet graft and 2) the larger the slits, the greater the scarring will be when it heals, and these scars will be permanent. Meshing serves two purposes: it allows blood and body fluids to drain from under the skin grafts, and because it is expanded, it allows the donor skin to cover a greater area. If possible, placing a graft as a sheet results in the least scarring and in the skin looking the most like non-injured skin.

Portions of this text courtesy: "Severe Burns" by Andrew M. Munster, M.D. and "Burn Care and Rehabilitation Principles and Practice" by Reginald L. Richard and Marlys J. Staley.

Chapter 40

Second Skins

Last spring [1996], a 68-year-old Northern California man suffered deep, third-degree burns when he dropped a cigarette and his pants leg caught fire. Unfortunately, such injuries are all too common. What's unusual is that this man became the first patient treated outside clinical trials with a new artificial skin that the Food and Drug Administration (FDA) had just approved for marketing the month before.

A serious burn is one of the most horrendous traumas the body can suffer. Every year, about 51,000 Americans are hospitalized for burn treatment, according to the American Burn Association, and 5,500 die. The good news is that the incidence and severity of burn injuries have declined significantly over the past 20 years. And patient survival keeps improving.

"This is a very exciting area," says Charles Durfor, Ph.D., in FDA's division of general and restorative devices. "Thirty to 40 years ago, many burn patients didn't live. Advances in treatment have created a whole new patient population that not only lives, but has an improving quality of life."

The first great strides were in getting patients through the initial shock, and preventing fluid loss. Controlling infection, a serious threat to burn patients, also improved. Specialized nutritional support has helped. Another leap occurred when doctors began surgically removing,

U.S. Food and Drug Administration, *FDA Consumer*, January-February 1997.

or excising, all burned tissue from the wound as soon as possible. After stabilizing the patient and cleaning out the wound, the next step is to cover it. "The sooner you close the wound, the sooner the patient gets better," says Robert Klein, M.D., medical director of the regional burn center at Children's Hospital Medical Center of Akron, Ohio.

"The problem is, we've never had an optimal way to do it," says Jerold Kaplan, M.D., director of the burn centers at Alta Bates Hospital in Berkeley, Calif., and at Children's Hospital in nearby Oakland. The need to cover wounds as quickly as possible while minimizing scarring and additional trauma has driven development of advanced wound dressings and skin substitutes. Kaplan treated the 68-year-old California man's wounds with Integra Artificial Skin Dermal Regeneration Template, from Integra LifeSciences Corp., Plainsboro, N.J. "Integra is a significant addition to the armamentarium of the burn surgeon," Kaplan says, and other surgeons agree.

Skin Deep

Surgeons also agree that no single product or technique is right for every burn situation. And so far, there's no true replacement for healthy, intact skin, which is the body's largest organ, and one of the most complex. It's the first line of defense against infection and dehydration, but it's more than just a physical barrier. Skin also helps control temperature through adjustments of blood flow and evaporation of sweat. It's an important sensory organ, too.

Skin thickness varies with age and body location, but averages only 1 to 2 millimeters (0.04 to 0.08 inches) thick. Thick or thin, it has two layers. The thin outer epidermis is nourished from the thicker, more sensitive dermis below. The outermost surface is a tough, protective coating of dead, flat, cells resembling paving stones. As these cells wear away, they're replaced from beneath. The innermost part of the epidermis consists of rapidly dividing cells, called keratinocytes, which produce keratin, a tough protein. Epidermis also contains a unique fatty substance that makes skin waterproof.

The skin's blood vessels, lymph vessels and nerves are in the dermis. Hair follicles, sweat glands, and oil glands also reside deep in this layer, which is mainly connective tissue. A network of collagen, the most common protein in the body, gives flexibility and structural support to the skin. Fibroblasts are the dominant cell type. Dermis plays a role in preventing wound contraction and scarring.

Treatment of burns depends on how deep and extensive they are, and the overall health of the patient. First-degree burns (such as sunburns) affect only the epidermis; they may peel but generally heal quickly. Second-degree burns damage the skin more deeply, causing blisters but sparing some of the dermal layer. Unless they're extensive, these burns usually heal without serious scarring. Third-degree burns destroy the full skin thickness, sometimes exposing muscle or bone, and require specialized treatment and skin grafts to obtain complete wound healing and reduce scarring. Left alone, the body tries to close wounds quickly by contraction, which results in serious scarring that is not only disfiguring, but can also be disabling.

Currently, the best wound covering most often is the patient's own skin. Healthy skin from another body site can be transplanted, which is called an autograft ("autos" means self). Sometimes little slits are cut so the resulting meshed graft can be stretched to cover more area. A split-thickness graft takes only the upper skin layer, and the donor site usually heals within several days. The thinner the graft, the faster the donor site heals. Surgeons may even take additional thin grafts from healed sites. Full-thickness grafts usually give a better-looking final result, but sometimes they don't adhere and survive. Donor sites are limited and autografting isn't always possible.

"People with great big burns don't have enough of their own skin, so you have to have some other way of covering them," says David M. Heimbach, M.D., director of the University of Washington Burn Center at Harborview, Seattle. Some patients can't withstand the additional trauma of a donor site wound. Older patients heal slowly and have thinner skin to begin with. And grafting creates another scar.

Doctors often use temporary coverings while patients get stronger, or while donor sites heal for additional harvesting. Two traditional possibilities are an allograft ("allos" means "other") of human skin, usually cadaver skin, or a xenograft ("xenos" means "stranger," in this case from another species) of pig skin. Cadaver skin is preferable, but as with other donated organs, sometimes it's in short supply and transmission of infectious agents is a concern. Human skin is regulated under FDA's Human Tissue Program, which requires donor screening for HIV (the AIDS virus) and hepatitis. In any case, the immune system rejects allo- and xenografts in a matter of days or weeks, and they must be removed and replaced. To avoid such problems, researchers and manufacturers are developing better wound dressings.

Advanced Dressings

FDA recognizes two broad categories of wound dressings—interactive and non-interactive. A variety of non-interactive dressings are available for covering first- and second-degree burns and other wounds. An interactive dressing is intended to actively promote wound healing by interacting directly with body tissues. Manufacturers must submit safety and effectiveness data to FDA in a pre-market approval application. FDA has approved two interactive wound dressings for use on third-degree burns: Integra Artificial Skin and Original BioBrane (Blue Label), marketed by Dow B. Hickam, Inc., New York.

BioBrane is a knitted nylon fabric bonded to an ultra-thin silicone rubber membrane coated with a protein (gelatin) derived from pig tissue. Clotting factors in the wound interact with the gelatin in the dressing, causing it to adhere to the wound within a day or so. The dressing remains in place until autografting becomes possible.

Integra is a two-layer membrane—a dermal layer that's a porous lattice of cross-linked collagen fibers, and a synthetic epidermal layer. The dermal layer acts as a biodegradable template that helps organize dermal tissue regeneration. Fibroblasts and other cells migrate into the lattice from surrounding healthy tissue, as do blood and lymph vessels. The fibroblasts degrade the temporary scaffold and recreate their own collagen matrix.

"The dermal part of the product is a permanent cover which the body converts into something which looks more like dermis than it looks like scar tissue," Heimbach says.

The outer synthetic layer provides the barrier functions of epidermis for two to three weeks; then the surgeon replaces it with a very thin autograft. "The ability to have the donor site be very thin and heal in just a few days is the big benefit," says Kaplan. "You're actually adding a procedure, but the end result is positive."

"It's a neat concept and it appears to work," says Heimbach, who has used Integra on more than 100 patients during clinical trials. He says the final results look much better than the alternative, meshed autografts. "We're excited about the new composite skin substitutes," he says.

Cultured Skin

Doctors prefer a thin graft to a thick one, but eliminating the donor site wound and scar altogether would be even better. That's done by growing the patient's skin in the lab, under special tissue culture conditions. Lab-grown skin products also have other potential uses for wounds other than burns, and for laboratory testing. From a postage stamp-size piece of skin, technicians can grow enough skin in about three weeks to nearly cover the body. Some medical centers are equipped for this sort of cell culture, and Genzyme Tissue Repair, Cambridge, Mass., does it as a commercial service. Cultured skin has been available for treating burns for about a decade, and in certain circumstances it can work well. "The problem here is you're putting on epidermis and not dermis," Kaplan says.

"Without both parts, you don't really have skin," Heimbach says. "You're grafting on scar tissue and that's not a satisfactory skin covering."

Less than 10 cells thick, it's also tricky to handle. "It's like gossamer," Kaplan says. And something has to cover the wound in the meantime. That's where Kaplan and others see a potentially useful combination. The patient's epidermis could be cultured during the two to three weeks while Integra's dermal layer becomes a suitable bed for grafting. "They're complementary," says Kaplan.

"You'd have the best of both worlds. You don't have any donor sites, and you have a good, durable, cosmetically acceptable cover," says Heimbach.

"Another approach we're actively working on is the one-step procedure," says Frederick Cahn, Ph.D., senior vice president, technology, Integra LifeSciences. The patient's own epidermal cells are isolated, as they would be for culturing, then seeded onto the dermal layer of Integra before it is applied to the wound. Both skin layers regenerate in place simultaneously, and only one surgical procedure is required. This procedure has worked well in animals, but hasn't been tried in humans yet.

Although physicians welcome new ways to help their patients, they're leery of "scar in a jar" products that might solve some problems while creating others. Last year, FDA held hearings on using the patient's own cells for structural repair in therapy, and heard a strong call for measures of efficacy. Based on the testimony presented, FDA has decided to regulate such therapy and is developing guidance documents to assist manufacturers in completing the premarket review process. "FDA recognizes that the area of tissue substitutes is a rapidly evolving area—and that medical and biochemical practice are also growing rapidly—and it's working aggressively to make sure it doesn't stifle development while continuing to ensure patient safety," says FDA's Durfor.

Investigators have developed other variations on cultured skin in the hope of providing off-the-shelf, living, temporary or permanent dressings. Clinical trials are under way testing them on burns and other wounds. For example, Advanced Tissue Sciences, La Jolla, Calif., developed its Dermagraft-TC skin replacement to be used as an alternative to cadaver skin for burns.

Treatment for burns keeps improving, but burn surgeons still have another important concern. "I think 95 percent of the burns we see are completely preventable," says Heimbach. He credits smoke detectors for a huge drop in the number of burns and deaths from house fires, but he hasn't seen much change in the number of accidents caused by carelessness or ignorance.

"The answer to the burn problem is prevention. Once it happens, it's too late," Klein says. "Be careful so you never need us."

Hope for Wounds That Won't Go Away

It may be hard for a healthy person to imagine having a wound that just won't heal, but that problem plagues millions of Americans. Non-healing wounds not only take an emotional toll, but also leave patients, their families, and society with a serious economic burden, ranging into billions of dollars.

The incidence of chronic wounds is far greater than burns and is expected to continue to increase as the population ages. Some of the treatment concerns are similar because the barrier function of skin is lost, putting the patient at risk for infection, and chronic wounds can be life threatening.

There are three general types of chronic wounds: pressure ulcers (bedsores or decubitus ulcers), venous ulcers, and diabetic ulcers. They have different causes, but the result is the same—localized tissue death. The factors that cause an ulcer to develop in the first place also interfere with healing. The cost per healed ulcer—when they heal at all—can climb into the tens of thousands of dollars, and as many as half recur within a year. Roughly three-quarters of a million American diabetics suffer with foot ulcers, which are responsible for more than 50,000 amputations a year.

Recent research efforts in pursuit of various growth factors to promote wound healing have been disappointing. Figuring out which growth factors to put in a wound—and when and at what dose—is a daunting, perhaps impossible, task. Some investigators have turned to cultured skin, arguing that applying cultured skin to wounds makes more sense than using growth factors because living cells already know how to produce growth factors at the right time and in the right amount.

Organogenesis Inc., of Canton, Mass., has developed Apligraf (formerly Graftskin), a two-layer living skin substitute derived from infant foreskins. The upper layer contains keratinocytes, the dominant cell type in the epidermis. The lower layer contains collagen and fibroblasts, the main constituents of dermis. Other cell types that trigger immunological response are absent, and, as a result, this engineered tissue is not rejected. Human trials of Apligraf for treating burns, diabetic ulcers, and for use in other skin surgeries are under way.

Cultured skin offers new hope for chronic wounds, but, as with burns, prevention is the best bet.

Skin Under Glass

In addition to its potential as an advanced wound dressing, cultured skin may also prove useful in laboratory testing. Many cosmetic, household product, pharmaceutical, and petrochemical companies are experimenting with cultured skin in the hope that in vitro (in glass, meaning in lab vessels) assays can replace or reduce animal testing for evaluating raw materials and final product formulations. FDA has long supported development of such methods, but the state of the science hasn't progressed yet to where it can fully replace animal testing, according to FDA's John Bailey, who heads the Office of Cosmetics and Colors in the agency's Center for Food Safety and Applied Nutrition.

Scientists can use isolated skin tissue to test skin penetration, irritation, toxicity, and other effects of various substances. Although cadaver skin works for some purposes, its uses are limited because the cells are dead. Cultured skin contains live, metabolizing cells that can better mimic how skin responds to various stimuli.

One example is the EpiDerm System, a model of human epidermis marketed by MatTek Corp., Ashland, Mass. Human-derived epidermal cells are grown under culture conditions that encourage formation of the characteristic cell subtypes and layers of epidermis. Another example is Skin2 , developed by Advanced Tissue Sciences, Inc., La Jolla, Calif. Some versions of Skin2 contain dermis as well as epidermis. These products are intended to be used for testing, not as dressings.

Lab-grown skin is used in two general ways. As a membrane to measure skin absorption, it doesn't work very well because it's much more permeable than skin, according to Robert L. Bronaugh, Ph.D., chief of the skin absorption and metabolism section in FDA's Office of Cosmetics and Colors. "A lot more work needs to be done before it can be used to simulate accurately the barrier properties of human skin," he says.

However, as an alternate test to measure irritation, cultured skin looks encouraging, according to Bronaugh. The U.S. Department of Transportation has approved the use of a Skin2 in vitro test kit as an alternative to animal testing of potentially corrosive materials. Although FDA wouldn't accept final safety data acquired from these in vitro assays, companies can use cultured skin in early screenings, and that saves animals, as well as money.

—by Carolyn J. Strange

Chapter 41

Scar Revision

The effect of facial scarring is more than skin deep. Often it is very difficult to evaluate the emotional impact of such injuries. This is especially true with children who are unable to verbalize their feelings about the scars, or in males who are taught to minimize their concern about their appearance. It is apparent that many people undergo unnecessary deformity because either they or their families have failed to deal with their concern over the effects of facial scarring or have failed to seek advice on what can be done to improve the appearance of facial scars.

The treatment of facial scarring can be the most gratifying thing that a facial plastic surgeon does. On the other hand, it would be unfair if we did not point out that it is also one of the most difficult and challenging aspects of this type of practice. Unlike most cosmetic procedures, incisions usually cannot be hidden. The area of incision has already been predetermined by the injury. Often it is in the worst possible place, such as on the cheeks or on the jaw line.

Timing Scar Revision

Patients tend to be impatient about the results of scar revision surgery. They are often already upset by the injury itself and find it

Howard A. Tobin, M.D., F.A.C.S., Facial Plastic & Cosmetic Surgical Center, reprinted from the website at www.newlook.com. © 2000; reprinted with permission.

difficult to understand that adequate and complete treatment may take many months or even several years.

Children and young adults are the most common victims of injury. Unfortunately, their skin tends to heal with more scarring as an accompaniment to their ability to heal more rapidly. Although these scars tend to fade with time, it still makes the treatment program more difficult. Furthermore, it makes it much more important to wait before initiating treatment since a scar that looks poor a month or so after injury may continue to greatly improve in appearance for many months. Ultimately, it may be so unnoticeable as to not require treatment.

Although the repair carried out at the time of injury does influence the amount of scarring that exists after healing, even the most careful repair may not provide a totally acceptable result. When treating the initial injury, one is never sure how tissues will heal. Lost tissue may have to be replaced with grafts. Wounds may have to be closed under tension. These are only some of the factors that tend to promote increased scarring.

Types of Treatment Available

Before instituting any form of treatment, we should watch the scar for a period of time. As long as there is significant improvement, then no surgical treatment should be instituted. Of course proper treatment at the time of and following injury, will help to minimize scarring. Instructions for wound care are available, on request, at the Center. Usually, within six months, the scar will have matured to near its optimum. If it is obviously unsatisfactory at that time, then scar revision should be considered.

Pressure and Massage: It is important to remember that sometimes conservative treatment is the best form of therapy. Repeated massage using cocoa butter or vitamin E can greatly improve the appearance of scars. In some cases, special pressure dressing may also be of use.

Cortisone Drugs: Various types of cortisone drugs may be used either as injections, topical preparations, or in the form of special tapes. These may well improve the scar to a point where surgery is not required.

Re-excision: In many cases, simple excision and re-closure of the wound will greatly improve the result. We may be able to close the wound without the tension that was present at the time of the initial repair. Furthermore, what was originally a jagged cut may now be changed into a clean surgical incision.

Zig-Zag-Plasty: The zig-zag-plasty is a technique of excising a scar and replacing the line with a geometric broken line. This type of wound tends to heal with less tension, and replaces a straight line scar with a broken line scar which tends to be less apparent to the eye. This is one of the most common and successful techniques of dealing with facial scars.

Dermabrasion or Laser Resurfacing: Dermabrasion is a surgical planing technique which can be used to smooth down raised or uneven scars. Most commonly used for acne scarring, it is frequently helpful in the treatment of other injury scars. More recently, the surgical laser has been found to be a superior resurfacing tool. Dermabrasion or laser resurfacing is frequently used as a planned component of the initial repair. Approximately five weeks after the initial wound is sutured, the repaired area is dermabraided. This often results in a scar less noticeable than it would have been without the combined dermabrasion.

Collagen Implantation: Collagen implantation involves the injection of a collagen material into the scar. It can be helpful in the treatment of depressed scars. In some cases, it can flatten the scars and make them almost imperceptible. Collagen does not result in permanent correction and treatment must be repeated after several months.

Silicone Pressure Therapy: In many cases, a silicone dressing can be applied to a raised scar and help to soften or thin out the scar. The mechanism of this effect is unknown at the present time, but it has proven useful in many cases. It is very safe and simple to use. The special silicone sheet is cut to size and applied to the scar. It should be kept in place for 12- to 24-hours-a-day, depending on tolerance. Effects are not immediate, but results are usually seen within several weeks.

Serial Excision: In many cases, wide or extensive scarring cannot be adequately treated with one operation. A planned, staged approach may be required in which several operations are utilized to lead to the best possible result. In some situations, a device called a tissue expander can be used to hasten this type of reconstruction.

Risks of Scar Revision

As mentioned, when dealing with scars, we must operate in the area predetermined by the accident. Most other cosmetic procedures involve the placement of scars in inconspicuous areas or areas that are known to heal with minimal scarring. Any time an incision is made, a scar will result. Unfortunately, the thickness and the texture of the scar is only partially related to the skill of the surgeon and the procedure itself. In no case will scar revision surgery eliminate a scar completely. In nearly all cases, it will minimize the scar. In very rare cases, the scar could be made worse. Although very uncommon, it is a risk that must be accepted by the patient.

For additional information contact: Howard A. Tobin, M.D., F.A.C.S., Facial Plastic & Cosmetic Surgical Center, 6300 Regional Plaza, Abilene, Texas 79606. (915) 695-3630; Toll Free (800) 592-4533; Fax (915) 695-3633; e-mail: n41gt@newlook.com.

Chapter 42

When Does Your Child Need a Plastic Surgeon?

Lacerations represent approximately 30-40 percent of all injuries that present to a pediatric emergency department (Gonzalez del Key & DiGiulio, 1997). The number of lacerations in children seen in the hospital emergency room is increasing (Knapp, 1997). The causative factors of these injuries are quite variable and may involve several areas of the body. After a systematic inventory of the wounds is made, the management of the injury(ies) is determined by the emergency room physician. Treatment of lacerations in children will be provided by the emergency room physician or a plastic surgeon can be consulted, however, parents often request that a plastic surgeon repair even small lacerations on the face.

Causation

The majority of the injuries in young children occur around the house, such as falling out of bed, off chairs, or down the stairs. In addition, there are those injuries occurring in the kitchen, backyard, basement, and while playing with toys. Automobile trauma occurs in sudden stops when the child is improperly restrained by a seatbelt or a car seat. The injuries usually have multiple areas of involvement. School accidents revolve around sports and outdoor recess play, with

"When Does Your Child Need a Plastic Surgeon? (Nursing Care of Trauma Patients)," by Joyce MacLean, in *Plastic Surgical Nursing*, Fall 1998, vol. 18, no. 3, p. 198(2). ©1998. American Society of Plastic and Reconstructive Surgical Nurses; reprinted with permission.

injuries incurred on the climbing apparatus, swings, or from running and falling.

With several million dogs present in the United States, there are frequent dog bites. Other causes of domestic injuries include falling around the swimming pool, playing with fireworks and guns, and lawnmower injuries. Serious accidents occurring on the farm include the avulsion of the scalp from long hair getting caught in tractor motors and other injuries caused by farm tools and machinery.

Wound Care

All wounds should be inspected for the degree of bleeding and possible communication with vital areas of the body, such as the brain, chest, and abdomen. An accurate description of areas, size, shape, and type of wound should be made and documented on the medical record. The wound itself is irrigated well with saline and all foreign bodies removed. If a fractured bone is suspected, x-rays should be obtained. Axial, coronal, and 3-D Cat Scans can assist with diagnosing a facial fracture.

For an aesthetically acceptable scar, there is more involved than the expert and careful placement of delicate sutures; great attention to detail must be taken to remove all foreign bodies in the wound. Gross debris should be removed, and wound edges should be unraveled before the final repair is undertaken. When they are available, temporary tacking sutures can be placed in the wound edges and a moist bulky dressing placed over the laceration as an initial treatment to reduce contamination from exposure.

When necessary, lacerations can wait for as long as 24 hours for final suturing, with minimal compromise of the end result if bleeding has been controlled and the wound has been cleansed (Vecchione, 1996). According to Dr. Kenneth Shaheen, of Troy, MI, "If the wound is well cleaned in an emergency room, a butterfly bandage can be applied and the wound can be sutured by the plastic surgeon in the office the next morning." However, it is unfortunate that patients often wait in the emergency room for a length of time before debris is removed from the wound. When the wound is finally attended to by the emergency room physician or the plastic surgeon, the opportunity for the optimal wound closure may have passed.

Consulting a Plastic Surgeon

The physician who performs the initial treatment and suturing of a laceration has the opportunity and the obligation to use sound techniques that result in normal healing (Vecchione, 1996). After the wound is assessed and cleaned and radiographs are obtained, it is the emergency room physician's responsibility to decide if it is appropriate to consult a plastic surgeon. Simple lacerations of the skin alone and not involving important structures are repaired by the emergency room physician, as long as he or she feels confident in repairing it. However, "Attempting to repair extensive soft tissue injuries of the face in a corner of the emergency room with inadequate light and without assistance invites frustration and second rate results. Such injuries should be repaired in the operating room with the help of at least a scrub nurse and a circulating nurse" (Shultz, 1997).

Major wounds involving fractures of facial bones and injury to essential anatomic structures of the face, such as facial nerves, lachrymal duets, and the inner canthal region of the eye are repaired by a plastic surgeon. "In deciding if a plastic surgeon should make the repair, the appearance of the wound must be considered," states Dr. Lauran Bryan of Royal Oak, MI. "Very few lacerations are clean, like a scalpel incision. They are usually bruising and crushing injuries, and we have to look at the tissue loss." Dr. Bryan said, "Lacerations with tissue loss that involve the lip, nose, and eyelid, especially if it involves the tarsal plate, should probably be repaired by the plastic surgeon."

Nursing Implications

Nursing assessment of all wounds including size, depth, shape, location, and bleeding should be recorded on the hospital record. In facial injuries, bleeding from the nose and mouth and distortion of tissue interfere with breathing. This type of obstruction of the airway can, at times, be handled by positioning, suctioning or placement of an oral airway.

Education should be provided for the parents and caregivers informing them that a plastic surgeon should be consulted only if there is a facial fracture or injury to the anatomic structures of the face. "Although we don't have an official policy regarding when a plastic surgeon is consulted, we do try to be sensitive to the wishes of the parents," says Heidi Shephard, Director of Emergency Center Nursing, William Beaumont Hospital. "If the parent insists, we will call a plastic surgeon, being sure to tell the parents that the plastic surgeon will bill the patient separately for the service." According to Dr. Shaheen, "The plastic surgeons are more likely to be 'over-called' for lacerations, rather than not be consulted when they should be." Support and comfort should be provided to the patient during treatment. Often a young child has to be restrained during suturing. This can cause high anxiety for both the caregiver and child. Explaining the need for restraints and providing support to the caregiver can alleviate some of this anxiety.

Patients are discharged home with a parent or caretaker. They receive written and verbal instructions concerning care of the laceration, pain management, and when to have sutures removed, in addition to any other pertinent instructions. They are encouraged to return to their pediatricians to have sutures removed. If the wound was sutured by the plastic surgeon, the sutures would be removed by him or her.

Gonzales del Rey, J.A., & DiGiulio, G.A. (1997). Wound care and the pediatric patient. In A.T. Trott (Ed.), *Wounds and lacerations*. St. Louis: Mosby-Year Book, Inc.

Knapp, J. F. (1997). What's new in pediatric emergency medicine? *Pediatrics in Review*, 18(12), 424-428.

Schultz, R.C. (1997). Soft tissue injuries of the face. In W.C. Grabb & J.W. Smith (Eds.), *Plastic Surgery* (5th Edition). Philadelphia: Lippincott-Raven Publishers.

Vecehione, T.R. (1996). Lacerations. In B.M. Barrett (Ed.), *Patient Care in Plastic Surgery* (2nd Edition). St. Louis: Mosby-Year Book, Inc.

Chapter 43

Prevention and Correction of Functional Tongue Defects

Total glossectomy (i.e., excision of the anterior and base of the tongue) procedures with laryngeal preservation are oncologically sound and result in acceptable oral function in postoperative patients. A study showed that 67% of patients who underwent total glossectomy procedures were able to swallow soon after surgery. The researchers also showed that an equivalent number of patients were able to swallow whether or not surgeons performed laryngeal suspensions. Patients without laryngeal suspensions, however, were more likely to have persistent aspiration problems. Two of 15 patients who did not undergo laryngeal suspensions required interval laryngectomy procedures for control of aspiration, whereas none of the 12 patients who underwent laryngeal suspension required laryngectomy procedures. None of the patients undergoing glossectomy procedures for salvage were long-term survivors; however, 67% of previously untreated patients survived 18 months, and 35% of previously untreated patients survived three years. All of these patients underwent tongue reconstruction procedures in which surgeons only used pectoralis major myocutaneous pedicle flaps.

Another researcher published a study that showed eight out of nine patients with preserved larynges and successful flap reconstructions of their tongues were able to have oral intake postoperatively. These

"Prevention and Correction of Functional Tongue Defects," excerpted from "Tongue Reconstruction Procedures for Treatment of Cancer" by John M. Truelson and Angela N. Pearce, in *AORN Journal*, March 1997, Vol. 65, No. 3., p. 534. © 1997 Association of Operating Room Nurses, Inc.: reprinted with permission.

patients' speech intelligibility ratings approached 85% to 90% by speech therapy evaluation, and eight out of 10 patients were decannulated after surgery. All patients underwent tongue reconstruction procedures with latissimus dorsi flaps (i.e., three patients underwent pedicle flap reconstructions, 12 patients underwent free flap reconstructions). Seven of the study's 15 patients still are alive after their treatments, with a posttreatment median of 22 months.

Another group of researchers studied patients who underwent glossectomy procedures with mandibular reconstructions in which eight of the study's 12 patients survived more than one year after surgery (i.e., six patients were able to eat pureed diets, two patients were able to take liquids). All eight patients were able to attain intelligible speech on objective examination by speech therapists. The other four patients died within one year and were incapable of intelligible speech or swallowing.

The same group of researchers later reported on 56 patients who underwent microvascular composite free flap procedures and compared the outcomes of immediate reconstruction procedures with secondary reconstruction procedures. Patients undergoing immediate reconstruction procedures were far more likely to be able to swallow and had superior speech results. Delayed tongue reconstruction procedures were not as successful because of scarring and irreversible damage of functional muscles involved in protecting the larynx. This underscores the importance of reconstructing the oral cavity immediately after glossectomy procedures.

Anterior Glossectomy Procedures

Surgeons use primary closure techniques when they repair anterior tongue defects of the lateral one fourth of the tongue. For hemiglossectomy procedures, surgeons may use flaps because the floor of the mouth often is resected in patients with tongue tumors. Radial forearm free flaps are used to repair this type of defect because they are very thin, pliable, and reliable.

Surgeons may use a technique that creates two lobes in the radial forearm flap to reconstruct the floor of the mouth and give bulk to the tongue with the same flap. This type of flap can give the tongue sensation either by neurorrhaphy procedures with a sensory nerve or by spontaneous reinnervation; however, this type of flap may add bulk to the tongue and limit the tongue's mobility. If the floor of the mouth is not involved in the surgical procedure, it can be sutured directly to the root of tongue if the genioglossus muscle is intact.

Total or subtotal glossectomy procedures of the anterior tongue result in the loss of all tongue mobility for articulation. Tongue reconstruction procedures, therefore, focus on building a mound of tissue so that the neotongue can push against the teeth and roof of the mouth for articulation. Surgeons also attempt to create a lingual sulcus (i.e., narrow groove in the oral cavity) for fitting dentures, although dental implants most often are required. Surgeons use radial forearm flaps for reconstruction of the total or subtotal glossectomy procedures. They pass the flap underneath the patient's mandible and suture it to the base of the tongue posteriorly and then fold the flaps to create a mound of tissue in the anterior portion of the patient's tongues. These flaps then can be folded and sutured to a patient's mandible to create a lingual sulcus.

The tongue falls back when its attachment to the anterior mandible is disrupted during tumor ablation. Surgeons solve this problem by suspending the hyoid and larynx from the mandible with permanent suture, which also brings the tongue forward. If the tongue tumor abuts but does not invade the mandible, the superior rim of the, mandible may be resected, leaving the arch intact (Figure 43.1.).

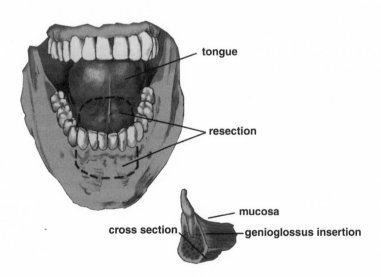

Figure 43.1. *Rim mandibulectomy. Teeth are removed en bloc with the dental alveolus. The tongue is held forward by the insertion of the genioglossus muscle. Resection of the genioglossus muscle requires suture suspension of the hyoid to the mandible. (Illustration by Mark Katmik Denver)*

243

If the full-thickness anterior arch of the mandible is resected with the tongue, the defect can be reconstructed with bone and skin free flaps from either the fibula, iliac crest, or scapula, The fibula has a smaller amount of skin available but is very reliable and easily contoured to fit the defect. The iliac crest free flap, however, gives an external skin paddle and an internal muscle reconstruction with the internal oblique, which cannot be mounded easily for tongue reconstruction. Radial forearm flaps and iliac crest free flaps have been used for reconstruction of combined tongue and mandible defects that have been removed surgically. Total defects of the tongue and mandible potentially can be reconstructed using iliac free flaps, but the two-flap design gives better oral reconstruction, mounding effects, and sensation.

Tongue Base Procedures

Tongue base resections can be reconstructed with any type of flap. The pectoralis major myocutaneous pedicled flap, radial forearm free flap, and lateral thigh flap techniques commonly are used at our institution (i.e., the University of Texas Southwestern Medical Center, Dallas). If the blood supply to the anterior tongue and the hypoglossal nerve can be preserved, then swallowing usually can be preserved for patients with strictly tongue base defects, regardless of the percentage of tissue surgeons resect. Hypoglossal nerve loss, however, usually causes significant problems for patients and prolongs their swallowing difficulties.

Total glossectomy procedures result in significant defects and difficulty swallowing regardless of what reconstruction technique surgeons use. Researchers recommend using latissimus dorsi or rectus abdominis flaps. Our surgeons use lateral thigh flaps for reconstruction of tongue base defects and combined anterior and tongue base defects. Lateral thigh flaps have greater bulk than other fasciocutaneous free flaps and they potentially can provide sensation to the tongue. Donor site function deficits do not occur because muscles are not resected. Surgeons do not resect patients' larynges even for total glossectomy procedures due to improved tongue reconstruction techniques. While aspiration is a concern, patients generally can handle their own secretions without aspiration. For those patients who are unable to swallow, gastrostomy procedures provide them a means for avoiding a total laryngectomy. Our surgeons reserve the use of total laryngectomy procedures for patients who have laryngeal involvement with cancer or intractable aspiration problems, but these procedures have not been necessary to date. Table 43.1 lists the alternative reconstructions for various defects.

Table 43.1. Free and Pedicle Flaps Used in Tongue Reconstruction Procedures

Donor Sites	Advantages	Disadvantages	Applications
Radial forearm	Thin, pliable tissue No sacrifice of muscle tissue	Tissue may be too thin Skin graft forearm necessary	Anterior tongue Floor of mouth
Lateral thigh	Bulkier than forearm tissue No muscle loss Large skin paddle	Difficult dissection	Total glossectomy Base of tongue Large defects
Latissimus dorsi	Bulky Covers large defects May retain bulk if innervated	Muscle loss Positioning difficult	Total glossectomy
Rectus abdominis	Bulky Covers large defects	Muscle loss Possible abdominal hernia	Total glossectomy Base of tongue
Fibula	Easy to contour No physiatric compromise	Skin paddle limited	Mandible, floor of mouth
Iliac crest	Skin and mucosal lining easy to contour	Shorter pedicle Possible abdominal hernia	Mandible, floor of mouth
Sacpula	Large skin paddle	Positioning difficult Difficult to contour	Mandible, floor of mouth

Chapter 44

Reconstruction of Ear Anomalies

Introduction

The Ear Anomalies Program at the Institute of Reconstructive Plastic Surgery at the New York University Medical Center emphasizes comprehensive, multidisciplinary care beginning at birth and continuing until the completion of facial growth. The team consists of specialists from plastic surgery, genetics, nursing, otolaryngology, prosthodontics, psychology, and speech pathology.

What is Microtia?

The term *microtia* indicates a small, abnormally shaped or absent external ear. It can be unilateral (occur on one side only) or bilateral (occur on both sides).

What is Aural Atresia?

The term *aural atresia* refers to the absence or incomplete formation of an external ear canal. Microtia is almost always accompanied by aural atresia. Patients with microtia and aural atresia do not have

The Microtia and Aural Atresia Division of the Institute of Reconstructive Plastic Surgery at New York University, reprinted from http://www.med.nyu.edu/PlasticSurg/Divs/micro.htm. © 1996, New York University Department of Plastic Surgery; reprinted with permission.

normal hearing on that side but may have completely normal hearing in the other ear.

Is Microtia an Isolated Problem?

In most patients microtia and aural atresia occur as an isolated condition. In some patients, however, the ear deformity occurs in conjunction with other facial deformities. The most common syndrome in which microtia accompanies other anomalies is called hemifacial microsomia which is a variable deformity that can involve the ear, the bones of the face, the fullness of the cheek tissue, and the function of the facial nerve. Another syndrome where microtia may be present is Treacher Collins syndrome. Because of the association with these syndromes, patients with microtia should be seen by a team of specialists and have a genetics evaluation so that the parents can be informed of any increased risk of these syndromes in future children.

What Should We Do if We Have a Child with Microtia?

The first priority during infancy is to ensure that there is sufficient hearing for language development. An accurate hearing test (audiogram) will be recommended as early as possible to establish the need for a hearing aid. There are two types of hearing tests, BAER testing (brain stem auditory evoked response testing) and behavioral testing. BAER testing is performed before the child is old enough to cooperate with behavioral testing. Reliable behavioral testing is the procedure of choice when the child is mature enough to cooperate. If the deformity is unilateral (occurs on one side only) and the opposite ear functions normally, a hearing aid will not be necessary. This is the case in the majority of patients.

What if Sufficient Hearing Does Not Exist?

If the deformity involves both ears, a hearing aid will be recommended immediately. Amplification needs (hearing aids) should ideally be met within the first few months of life. Surgery to restore hearing may not be recommended for several years.

How Often Should Hearing and Language be Monitored?

Regular monitoring of hearing and language is critical and should be performed at least as often as outlined in the protocol below.

Do Patients with Miocrotia/Aural Atresia Require Any Other Tests?

We recommend a high-resolution, three-dimensional Computed Tomography (CT) scan of the temporal bones at approximately age five in order to rule out a benign tumor of the middle ear known as a cholesteatoma, which is more common in aural atresia patients. In addition, the CT scan will indicate if the middle ear structures are adequate for surgical reconstruction of the external auditory canal. While all patients are candidates for reconstruction of the external ear, not all patients are candidates for reconstruction of the canal and middle ear.

If Surgery is Recommended to Reconstruct the Ear Canal, When is it Performed?

It is performed after the age of six and is coordinated with the surgical reconstruction of the external ear. It is important that the first stages of external ear reconstruction be performed prior to reconstruction of the ear canal.

At What Age is the External Ear Reconstruction Initiated?

This depends on the patient's size and maturity but generally occurs after the age of six years.

How Many Stages Are Required to Reconstruct An Ear?

The outer ear reconstruction usually involves three-to-four stages. In the first stage, a cartilage framework is carved from pieces of rib cartilage and inserted under the skin on the side of the head where the new ear will be. This procedure takes approximately four hours and requires a general anesthetic and a two-day hospital stay. The second, third, and fourth stages are short, "touch-up" type procedures which, in some patients can be performed on an outpatient basis. Because of the patient's age they usually require a general anesthetic, but in older patients can be performed under local anesthesia. In the second stage the earlobe is rotated into the correct position. The third stage involves deepening of the conchal bowl (the central part of the ear) and construction of the tragus. In the final stage a skin graft is inserted behind the ear to lift it off the head so that it more closely resembles a normal ear.

Who are the Members of the Microtia Team?

The microtia team consists of medical and surgical specialists who evaluate and manage all aspects of the child's condition. The plastic surgeon directs the team and will perform all necessary external ear reconstruction. The audiologist evaluates the child's hearing. The nurse specialist is the liaison between patient/family and other members of the team. He/She provides information and support to new families, as well as pre- and post-operative teaching. The otolaryngologist evaluates and manages any abnormalities of the middle or inner ear, and performs the canalplasty surgery (the procedure which will create an ear canal if it is indicated). The patient services representative assists families with issues such as insurance, fees, coordination of appointments, travel arrangements, and financial support. In some patients an artificial ear is recommended and is made by a prosthodontist. The psychologist performs psychometric testing and is available for counseling and referral to community mental health resources. The speech pathologist evaluates the quality of speech and language development and recommends speech therapy as needed.

What Other Support Is Available?

It is often difficult for parents to deal with their own responses to their child's condition, in addition to the responses of other people. Forward Face (800- 422-FACE), founded at the Institute of Reconstructive Plastic Surgery, is a self-help group consisting of patients and families affected with facial birth defects and is a helpful resource for families with these concerns.

Protocol for Audiologic Testing

I. Bilateral (both right and left sides) aural atresia

A. An audiogram is recommended within the first few days of life prior to discharge from the hospital. The test is repeated until consistent, reliable results are obtained.

B. An audiogram is then performed every three months until age two and then every six months until age four.

C. All patients with bilateral microtia require amplification (bone conduction hearing aids) within the first few months of life.

D. A speech evaluation is recommended as soon as the child is fitted with a hearing aid. Patients with bilateral atresia may require speech therapy as often as 2 to 3 times per week for the first three years of life.

II. Unilateral (one side) aural atresia

A. An audiogram should ideally be performed within the first few days of life prior to discharge from the hospital.

B. The test is repeated every three months until age two, and then every six months until age four. In the event of a problem such as an infection in the normal ear, more frequent audiograms may be recommended.

C. In general, patients with unilateral atresia do not require a hearing aid unless problems develop in the unaffected ear, or language/learning difficulties exist in the early stages of development.

D. A speech evaluation is performed within the first two months of life and is repeated at six-month intervals. Some unilateral patients may require speech therapy as the localization of sounds is a potential problem.

Chapter 45

Breast Cancer Network Update: Breast Reconstruction

Breast reconstruction surgery has become so refined that it can be accomplished on almost every woman who has had a mastectomy. Today, about a third of those who have a breast removed choose to have it rebuilt using autologous tissue (their own tissue) or reconstructed with an implant. Most implants are circular silicone envelopes filled with saline or silicone gel or both.

Even women who have a lumpectomy (removal of the cancer and a small amount of surrounding breast tissue) may benefit from reconstruction if so much breast tissue has been excised that the breast is much smaller than the opposite one. However, there are several shortcomings of reconstruction after lumpectomy. For one, lumpectomy is usually followed with a course of radiation therapy, and tissue that has been irradiated has more difficulty healing. Also an implant behind the breast may not restore the post-lumpectomy breast contour very well, since the tissue is missing in only one area. At this time, there is no such thing as an implant the size and shape of tissue removed in a lumpectomy.

Reconstructive surgery can be done immediately after a mastectomy (immediate reconstruction) or some time after healing from the mastectomy is complete (delayed reconstruction). Some women and their doctors prefer immediate reconstruction, because it may lessen the emotional impact of the mastectomy. However, when both mastectomy

American Cancer Society, "Breast Cancer Network Update—Breast Reconstruction." Reprinted from http://www.cancer.org. © 1997, American Cancer Society; reprinted with permission.

and reconstruction are done at the same time, the operation is longer and there is an increased chance of wound healing problems. So you and your doctors will have to weigh that risk against the benefits for you. In general, if chemotherapy is part of the treatment plan, surgeons are more likely to recommend delayed reconstruction, particularly if more aggressive types of chemotherapy are planned. They also take into account the size and location of the cancer, which determines the amount of skin to be removed in the mastectomy as well as other health factors such as age and obesity and whether the woman smokes or has diabetes.

The goal of this surgery is to create a breast that matches the opposite breast. Occasionally that requires reducing the size of the opposite, healthy breast—especially in women with very large breasts—or inserting an implant to enhance a smaller breast. In some cases, a woman may find a breast lift of the healthy breast gives her a more balanced, symmetrical contour.

Women who are pleased with the results of breast reconstruction—and most who have it are satisfied—say the procedure helped counter some of the negative effects that mastectomy had on their sense of well-being and their feelings about their femininity and sexual desirability. In making the decision to have the operation, they considered practical aspects, such as not wanting to wear a prosthesis and having more freedom in choosing clothing, as well as emotional concerns, such as wanting to feel less sexually inhibited. Whatever motivated the desire for breast reconstruction, studies show that most women are happy with the results, even when several operations are necessary to achieve a natural appearing breast.

But reconstruction isn't for everyone. Women who choose not to have reconstruction feel just as comfortable with their decision as those who do have the surgery. Women who reject reconstruction say they simply don't want additional surgery, and sometimes multiple procedures. They believe reconstruction presents too many risks or is too frightening and that nothing really replaces a breast. Some fear there will be complications. And some say no because they feel comfortable wearing the breast prosthesis. In many ways, breast reconstruction is merely an internal prosthesis. In general, older women are less likely to have reconstruction, since it involves more operative time and more complications because they are older.

As with any surgery, it's important to get at least one other opinion about the method and timing of your reconstructive surgery. It's also helpful to talk to other women who have had reconstructive surgery. They can discuss their own experience with the benefits and drawbacks of reconstruction. The American Cancer Society's Reach to Recovery program can help you arrange a meeting with a woman who has had the surgery that you are contemplating.

Research indicates that most women know at the time of their cancer surgery whether they want reconstruction. This is good, because it enables you to enlist a plastic surgeon as part of the treatment team and incorporate his or her opinion into treatment decisions. Something as basic as the placement of the incision for an open biopsy can have an impact later if a mastectomy followed by reconstructive surgery is needed. However, if you don't know whether you want to undergo this additional surgery, it's better to wait. In fact, for some women it's better to postpone the decision. Women who have a delayed reconstruction actually know what living with a mastectomy is like and have made a decision, based on that knowledge, to have a reconstruction. Those who have an immediate reconstruction never know if they would have been comfortable living with the appearance of a mastectomy. Some women undergo the surgery years after mastectomy.

At the moment, insurance coverage for breast reconstruction is very uncertain. Some companies cover the initial procedure, but not the operations that are needed to refine the results. Be sure to check with your insurer before making your final decision. And be aware that the costs can vary greatly; if there are complications, the hospital bill can be as much as $15,000 to $20,000.

Breast Implants

The oldest and simplest method of reconstructing the breast is to create a mound with a synthetic implant. The surgeon inserts the implant through the mastectomy incision and under the pectoralis major (chest) muscle. Occasionally, the surgeon may insert the implant through a new incision on the side of the breast nearest the armpit.

Many different size implants and some slightly differently shaped ones are available today. Each type has advantages and disadvantages. From an appearance point of view, women with small to medium, rounded breasts have the best result with implants matching the opposite breast.

Types of implants: There is some controversy about the safety of silicone gel implants. Many women prefer them to saline-filled implants because the silicone feels more like breast tissue, and the gel shifts with movement more naturally. However, if a leak occurs, saline is absorbed into the body and is harmless. There has been a question whether silicone can trigger certain connective tissue and auto immune conditions (diseases in which the body's immune system attacks normal tissues). In 1992 the Food and Drug Administration restricted the use of silicone implants in order to study the question. Those who desired reconstruction with silicone-filled implants after mastectomy were given access to clinical trials. Studies completed thus far have failed to show an increased risk of auto-immune disease among women with silicone implants. As a result, several organizations, including the American Cancer Society, have petitioned the FDA, to ease the restrictions. In fact, other countries did not take silicone implants off the market and the situation that occurred in the United States may be a reflection of our unique medical-legal climate.

Implant surgery: Regardless of the type of implant, the actual surgery to insert it is relatively simple. When done at the time of a mastectomy, the reconstruction adds only about a half hour to an hour to the surgery. There are drains in place, and recovery time is longer due to the additional surgery, but the care afterward is the same as for mastectomy alone. Delayed reconstruction requires about an hour and half. Drains are not routine, and recovery is much quicker than it is after immediate reconstruction because the mastectomy wound has already healed.

Tissue expanders: The surgeon usually inserts a temporary tissue expander under the pectoralis muscle to stretch the muscle and the skin over the chest wall. The tissue expander is a silicone envelope with a valve-like opening or port through which a small amount of saline is injected. Every week or two for one to three months saline is injected until the expander is inflated to a size slightly larger than the implant will be. This stretching is painless just like the stretching of the abdomen that occurs with pregnancy.

Once these tissues are able to accommodate an implant and allow for a natural droop of the breast, the surgeon will replace the expander with a permanent implant. This is a 30-minute operation that can be done on an outpatient basis. Usually general anesthesia is used, but no overnight stay is required.

Some surgeons prefer an implant that combines the expander with the permanent implant. After the skin expansion is complete, the filling valve is sealed, and the expander remains in the breast as a permanent implant. The disadvantage of this particular type of implant is that the valve, which remains in place, may leak. Also, sometimes a slightly different shaped implant must be inserted for the permanent implant.

Complications and side effects of implants: As with any surgery, there is a risk of postoperative complications such as infection, seroma (accumulation of fluid in the surgical wound), and bleeding. In the case of reconstruction, these problems also include a loss of sensation in the breast; movement of the implant; breast asymmetry, or difference in the size and/or shape of the breasts; and extrusion, in which the implant begins to push out through the healing incision. The most common complication is a phenomenon known as capsular contraction, in which the pocket of scar tissue that forms around the implant becomes abnormally hard and can contract over the implant, causing the reconstructed breast to be misshapen.

Latissimus dorsi flap: If there is not enough skin to cover the implant, if the muscle over the chest wall has been removed, or if the skin has been so damaged by radiation that it cannot be stretched, the surgeon will remove a fan-shaped section of muscle and skin from the back attached to a portion of tissue, called a pedicle. The pedicle remains intact and contains the blood supply of the flap. This latissimus dorsi flap, which is named for the back muscle from which it comes, is tunneled under the skin and pulled out through an opening in the chest. It is then sutured in place over the mastectomy site. The surgeon then places an implant under the muscle to complete the reconstruction.

The latissimus dorsi flap procedure is obviously a much more complicated operation than an implant insertion. There is a scar on the woman's back, and there is a potential for shoulder problems because a portion of the muscle governing range of motion to the shoulder has been removed. There is about a 2-percent risk that a portion of the flap will not heal properly, and another operation may be necessary. However, this procedure usually creates a better result than when an implant is used alone, particularly in women with large breasts, or in women after radiation.

Autologous Reconstruction of the Breast

Several techniques exist for using the body's own tissue to build a mound that feels and appears like a natural breast. The most common technique—the TRAM flap—carries its own blood supply. Another method—the free flap—requires meticulous and difficult microsurgery to connect tiny blood vessels in the flap to those in the chest wall.

TRAM Flap: The TRAM (transverse rectus abdominous muscle) flap uses tissue taken from the woman's abdomen. The surgery is complicated and time-consuming, adding many hours to a mastectomy operation when the reconstruction is immediate.

A section of skin, underlying fat, and a portion of abdominal muscle is excised, leaving one or two pedicles of tissue with the natural blood supply. The flap is tunneled under the abdominal wall to the chest and rotated to fit the mastectomy wound. The edges of the breast incision are sutured to the flap.

Along with creating a breast with a natural texture, the technique also give the stomach a flatter appearance. However, some doctors caution against thinking of this as a tummy tuck, as there are side effects not normally associated with that cosmetic procedure. (For instance, some women experience abdominal weakness, sometimes to the point of being unable to do a sit-up). There is also an increased risk for developing an abdominal hernia (bulging of internal tissues through an area of weakness in the abdominal muscles and connective tissues). The TRAM flap can be sculpted to create a shape to match the other breast instead of just the typical round shape of an implant.

The TRAM flap procedure is major surgery that requires a week in the hospital and another four to six weeks or longer of recovery at home. Women who smoke cannot have this operation; they are likely to develop healing problems because smoking causes deterioration of the blood vessels. Although this operation is performed more than tissue expanders for women after radiation, they do have a higher rate of complications. In these women, fresh, unirradiated tissue is brought into the breast area. Women with abdominal scars or women without enough abdominal fat are not candidates for the surgery.

Free Flap: This is sometimes called a free TRAM because an island of fat and skin is removed from the abdomen. However, rather than leaving a pedicle attached to a blood supply, the entire island is cut "free" and stitched in place to the mastectomy wound. A surgeon who specializes in microsurgery attaches the blood vessels supplying the flap to those in the chest wall. Since it's not necessary to remove as much muscle from the abdomen, the side effects of the TRAM muscle removal, including abdominal hernia, should be avoided.

A free flap graft can also be made from the soft tissue, muscle and skin of the buttocks. This gluteal free flap is performed when other options are not possible. It may cause hip problems, the sciatic nerve may become injured causing leg pain, numbness, and weakness, and it is technically more difficult to accomplish than the free TRAM procedure.

Complications: Autologous breast reconstruction is major surgery that can require several hours in the operating room. The immediate complications are those associated with any operation—such as infection, formation of blood clots in the legs (which is why you will be encouraged to move about in bed after surgery and get out of bed the next day), and accumulation of blood and/or fluid in the breast or donor site that must be drained.

Much more likely, though still not common, are complications in healing. If the blood supply is not adequate, the skin over the reconstructed breast may not heal properly and will die, requiring another operation to replace it. Sometimes, too, fatty tissue degenerates and causes a thickening that can be painful and feels similar to a lump or tumor, which can be very frightening. The surgeon will take a biopsy of the thickening to check for cancer cells. Fluid or blood may continue to accumulate and must be withdrawn through a needle or the surgeon may insert a drain that allows the liquid to exit the body.

Nipple-Areola Reconstruction

In order to give the breast a realistic appearance, many women choose to have the nipple and surrounding areola reconstructed also. There are several techniques used to accomplish this, but usually tissue from heavier skin from the upper inner thigh is used. (Labial tissue is not used.) Some tissue from just under the skin can create nipple projection. When healing is complete, the areola can be tattooed with a flesh-colored pigment. This refinement procedure is most often done after the reconstructed breast has healed completely.

Chapter 46

The Surgery: Deciding about Breast Implants for Reconstruction

When thinking about surgery for breast cancer you will have many important decisions to make. One decision is whether to have surgery for breast reconstruction at all. As expected, women have different opinions and views about reconstruction.

A few reasons why some women decide **FOR** reconstruction with breast implants:

- to restore body image following mastectomy surgery for breast cancer,
- to replace an external breast form (prosthesis),
- to avoid being constantly reminded of their breast cancer diagnosis,
- to avoid embarrassment in public dressing areas, and
- to help create a look that makes them feel more comfortable with or without clothes.

A few reasons why some women decide **AGAINST** reconstruction with breast implants:

- they understand that breast implants are not lifetime devices, that they may have to undergo multiple surgeries and they want to avoid more surgery,

U.S. Food and Drug Administration, Office of Consumer Affairs, reprinted from www.fda.gov/oca/breastimplants/bitac.html, revised/posted 12/7/98.

- they feel the risks of surgery and anesthesia are greater than the benefits,

- they are concerned about potential known and unknown risks from breast implants for themselves and their children should they become pregnant,

- they feel they are able to adjust to a new body image without reconstruction with breast implants, and

- they prefer to wear an external breast form (prosthesis).

If you decide on breast reconstruction, there are currently two surgical techniques:

- **The "flap" technique.** This surgery rebuilds the contour of the breast by taking tissue from other areas of the body. The TRAM (transverse rectus abdominis musculocutaneous) flap technique may be used to reconstruct one or both breasts at the same time. The flap technique involves moving skin, muscle and fat to the breast area from the abdomen, back, or buttock to rebuild the breast. There will be a scar in the area where the flap was lifted. The flap technique is considered a major operation and, for medical reasons, is not suitable for everyone. This, like all operations, should be discussed carefully with your doctor. In some cases, breast implants may be used in addition to the flap procedure.

  It is important to note that the TRAM flap operation can be done only once. The TRAM flap can be used to reconstruct one or both breasts, but only in one operation. If the TRAM flap is used to reconstruct one breast, and a mastectomy is later required on the other breast, reconstruction of the second breast must be done through other means (i.e., insertion of a breast implant).

- **Insertion of breast implants.** The surgeon inserts the implant into a pocket created under the skin. The pocket may be located either behind (submuscular) or in front (submammary) of the chest muscle.

Ask your doctor about the pros and cons of each implant technique. If you decide to have reconstruction for one breast, you may need to think about surgery on the other breast to achieve a similar appearance.

Special Concerns for Women with Breast Cancer

Here are some of the known risks or problems with breast implant surgery for women with breast cancer:

- The physical and cosmetic results with breast implants may be affected by chemotherapy, radiation therapy, or any other factor which significantly alters the healing process.

- Skin necrosis (dying skin) may occur because circulation to the remaining tissue has been changed by a mastectomy or other trauma to the breast area. Also, skin necrosis may be increased as a result of radiation treatment.

- It usually takes more than one operation to achieve the desired cosmetic outcome, especially if this procedure includes rebuilding the nipple.

Timing for Reconstruction with Breast Implants

Reconstruction can be done either at the time of breast cancer surgery or at a later date. If breast surgery and implant surgery are done at the same time, the surgeon usually uses the same incision to insert the implant. Another option is to insert a temporary tissue expander. In this case, in a second operation after the skin has stretched sufficiently, the surgeon will remove the expander and replace it with an implant. Another option is to insert the implants at some time after the mastectomy. With delayed insertion, the surgeon may still be able to use the mastectomy or lumpectomy scar to insert the implant. The surgeon should discuss with you which approach is the most desirable for you, and the associated risks.

Recreation of the Nipple and Areola following Reconstructive Surgery

After your breast has healed from the original implant surgery, you may want your nipple and areola (darker skin around the nipple) rebuilt. This procedure can usually be performed on an out-patient basis. Ask your surgeon to explain the various ways this can be done.

Your Expectations—Reconstruction or Augmentation

Your consideration of breast implants, for reconstruction or for augmentation, should be based on realistic expectations of the outcome.

To help you get an idea of what results may be possible, look at before and after pictures of patients who have had this surgery. Your doctor may have some to show you. You may also want to talk with other women who have had this surgery at least a year before with the same surgeon. Keep in mind, however, that there is no guarantee that your results will match those of other women.

Your results will depend on many individual factors, such as your overall health; chest structure and body shape; healing capabilities (which may be hindered by radiation and chemotherapy, smoking, alcohol and various medications); bleeding tendencies; prior breast surgery(ies); infection; skill and experience of the surgical team; the type of surgical procedure; and, the type and size of implant.

Scarring is a natural outcome of surgery, and your doctor will try to keep scars as subtle as possible. She or he can explain the location, size, and appearance of the scars you can expect to have. For most women, scars will fade over time to thin lines, although the darker your skin, the more prominent the scars are likely to be. Usually the body will develop a fibrous capsule which can be thick or thin around the implant which is a normal physiologic response to a foreign object in the body.

It is important to remember that implants age over time and may need to be replaced. Although your implant may last for many years, you should not expect it to last indefinitely.

General Description of the Surgery

Breast implant procedures can be performed on an outpatient (not hospitalized) basis or at a hospital. Breast implant surgery can be done under local anesthesia or under general anesthesia.

Breast implant surgery can last from one to several hours depending on whether the implant is inserted behind or in front of the chest muscle, and whether surgery is performed on one or both breasts. Prior to surgery, the doctor should discuss with you the extent of surgery, the estimated time it will take, and the choice of drugs for pain and nausea.

Postoperative Recovery

The doctor should describe to you the usual postoperative recovery process, the possible complications that can arise, and the expected recovery period. Following the operation, as with any surgery, some pain, swelling, bruising, and tenderness can be expected, but they should disappear with time.

Medications for pain and nausea can be prescribed. Some women may experience fever, bleeding or other symptoms of infection; these should be reported immediately to the doctor. Patients should be instructed about wound healing and appropriate wound care.

If the surgery is done in a hospital, the length of the hospital stay will vary according to the type of surgery, the development of any postoperative complications, your general health, and the type of coverage your insurance provides.

Follow-Up

Ask your surgeon about follow-up care, including a schedule of follow-up examinations, advice about limitations to your activities, precautions you should take, and when you can return to your normal routine. (If you are enrolled in a clinical trial, your surgeon should give you a schedule for follow-up exams set by the study plan.)

Chapter 47

The Psychological Outcome of Breast Reconstruction

My first experience with breast cancer as a nurse was in 1974. I was a 23-year-old nursing student and working as an operating room technician. A radical mastectomy was being performed on a 52-year-old woman. As I passed clamps and scissors to the two surgeons, I struggled to conceal the shock I was experiencing. "Is it really necessary to remove so much tissue for such a small lump?" "Yes," the doctor replied, "It's either this or she'll die."

It was 10 years later, but I would begin my work with patients undergoing breast reconstruction. During the 7-1/2 years that I worked as an operating room supervisor and assistant to a plastic surgeon. I responded to the needs of a number of women during their time of crisis. We would see each other every week or two for a year, becoming friends, and treatment would come to an end. Their lives would go on, and I would continue my work with a new patient, then another and another.

My work with reconstruction patients continues as Patient Informational Coordinator for Mentor H/S, a breast implant manufacturer. Hundreds of women who have had breast cancer call me each year. I provide information, answer questions, and help educate.

Etched in my memories are emotion-filled faces and voices of shock, fear, confusion, sorrow, and resignation followed by acceptance.

"The Psychological Outcome of Breast Reconstruction." (Special Issue on Breast Reconstruction), by Diane Hart. *Plastic Surgical Nursing*, Fall 1996 vol. 16, no. 3, pg. 167(5). ©1996, American Society of Plastic and Reconstructive Surgical Nurses; reprinted with permission.

Individual women of various lifestyles and personalities as well as different levels of financial and social status, all have one thing in common—breast cancer, mastectomy, decisions, and reconstruction. Many were experiencing an interruption in their lives, a stress on their relationships and a drain on their finances. But the even greater challenge they faced was the life and death crises of an illness that is both life threatening and disfiguring.

Researchers such as Schain, Goldberg and Kasper have documented the psychosocial effects of breast-loss on women and their relationships (Schain, 1991; Goldberg, Stoltzman, & Goldberg, 1984; Kasper, 1995). Jones, Matheson, and Rowland looked at psychological adjustment, counseling needs and patient's response to their altered body image (Jones & Reznikoff, 1989; Matheson & Drever, 1990; Rowland Holland, Chaglassian, & Kinner, 1993). The alternation of body image first occur with mastectomy and continues with reconstruction. Goin, Cederma and Wellisch provide insight into the effects of various types of reconstruction (Goin & Goin, 1988; Cederna, Yates, Chang, Cram, & Ricciardelli, 1995; Wellisch, Schain, Noone, & Little, 1987).

The following article is a compilation of my personal experience, and excerpts from literature presented as an overview of the psychological effects of mastectomy and reconstruction.

As with any body part amputation, the loss of a breast can have devastating effects on a woman. The more she values her breasts the greater will be the effect on her self-image (Goldberg, et al., 1984). Difficult choices have to be made to assure health and preserve appearance (Goldberg et al., 1984). Mastectomy can affect all areas of a woman's life and produce significant psychological challenges. Negative perceptions of body image can increase self-consciousness.

In coming to terms with their loss, mastectomy patients experience psychological reactions similar to those coping with death and dying:

1. denial;
2. rage—anger and frustration;
3. depression and despair;
4. acceptance or non-acceptance.

Pseudo-acceptance may be a reaction experienced by the stoic patient who heals quickly on a physical and emotional level. This reaction may mask deeper feelings of loss, helplessness and depression (Matheson & Drever, 1990).

Women learn to cope with their breast cancer and mastectomy in very individual ways. Having a preexisting positive self-image provides a basis for greater tolerance of distress, while a negative self-concept may exacerbate feelings of inadequacy.

Married Women

There is a strong need to involve the patient's significant other in the reconstructive process. Open communication and counseling should be encouraged to help them deal with their tears. Reassurance from the spouse helps the patient not to feel alone and restores her morale (Goldberg et al., 1984). The spouse's reaction may also influence how the woman views herself and her choice regarding breast reconstruction (Schain, Jacobs, & Wellisch).

In a study by Matheson and Drever (1990) many husbands said that the absence of one or both breasts was acceptable to them. Others may experience a sense of loss and be unable to clearly express their feelings. In Matheson and Drever's study, many husbands did not feel a need for their wives to have more surgery and relayed their fears of additional surgery. Thirty-four percent were mildly to strongly opposed to reconstruction, 33% were in favor of reconstruction, and 33% were neutral (Matheson & Drever, 1990). Another study of husbands surveyed by Memorial Hospital reported 17% were negative towards reconstruction and unwilling to understand their wives' desire for reconstruction (Schain et al.).

Reintegration of sexual identity is facilitated with time. Generally speaking, sexual relationships that were good before the cancer and mastectomy will continue to be good afterwards (Schain et al.) and may even he strengthened by the crisis. Likewise, couples who were emotionally supportive of each other before will usually be emotionally available afterwards.

Single Women

Unmarried women have additional burdens. They tend to have greater financial problems, and increased difficulty with body image and social adjustment. Lack of a significant other to provide comfort or support can increase a sense of loneliness. During the process of reconstruction the woman may need to share her feelings with others. Often accompanying this is the need for approval for choosing reconstruction and validation that the new breast is acceptable.

Some women may avoid new relationships. Anxiety over disclosure and feelings of disfigurement could lead to coping mechanisms such as avoidance. Negotiation techniques may be used in an effort to delay a level of intimacy that neither are ready to manage (Schain et al.). In a new relationship, the reality of the mastectomy and the uncertain future, may be something some men would rather not handle (Kasper, 1995).

Support Network

The patient's environment and support network is the best indicator of how well she will be able to adjust to breast cancer. A woman's spouse, family, friends, and medical personnel can either positively or negatively influence a woman's self-image and state of mind. Since there is a strong family pattern to breast cancer, there is a significant possibility that other family members have had mastectomies. If one chooses reconstruction and the other has not, feelings of jealousy may arise (Schain et al.). The decisions the patient chooses regarding breast reconstruction may be influenced by the reactions of her relatives.

Another important factor is the development of a professional support network. This can be facilitated by the doctor and the nurse by providing information to the patient regarding professional organizations. The patient's existing support structure should be evaluated and then supplemented with additional avenues. Literature should be provided to the patient that details education and treatment choices available. A list of cancer support organizations and their phone numbers should be made available, such as:

- The American Cancer Society;
- American Society of Plastic and Reconstruction Surgeons (ASPRS);
- National Breast Cancer Coalition;
- National Organization for Women;
- Susan G. Komen Foundation; and
- Y-Me Breast Cancer Support Program.

Reconstruction: A Woman's Choice

A patient's decision on whether or not to have reconstruction surgery is usually based on five factors:

1. self-knowledge;
2. economics;
3. medical choices and safety;
4. self-determined needs; and
5. interpersonal relationships (Schain et al.).

Increased knowledge helps a woman to explore her motives for reconstruction and her resistances. Motives that generally influence her decision to reconstruct are to:

1. be able to wear more styles of clothes;
2. eliminate external prosthesis;
3. be less preoccupied with physical self;
4. feel more balanced;
5. feel "whole" again;
6. feel more feminine;
7. be less preoccupied with cancer; and
8. improve marital or sexual relations.

There are many references throughout the literature that discuss the benefits of reconstruction. These benefits include enhanced body image, a sense of femininity, psychological well-being, and self-confidence about their appearance. Many women report improvement in their personal and intimate relationships, while others cite a healing effect from reconstruction.

Sloan Kettering Hospital in New York surveyed 83 women seeking breast reconstruction. When measuring satisfaction with their surgical outcome, 83% were satisfied with their overall results (i.e., size, shape, nipple, and symmetry), 12% were dissatisfied and 5% were neutral. The women in this study said they were motivated to have reconstruction because of the negative outcome of mastectomy and the aggravation with wearing a prosthesis. These women scored high on self-esteem and felt they had the right to improve their discomfort and physical defect. They pursued reconstruction, often overcoming obstacles and a lack of emotional support.

Immediate or Delayed Reconstruction

The question more and more today is not whether to reconstruct but when is the optimal time to reconstruct. Concerns focus in two areas: (1) medical safety, and (2) psychological impact.

Mounting evidence indicates immediate reconstruction has positive value. By reconstructing immediately, the woman avoids the embarrassment of changing breast size. Thus, she is spared some of the pain and distress of breast loss. The psychological needs of the patient should be evaluated and then utilized to determine the appropriate timing for reconstruction.

Various factors may cause some women to delay reconstruction. They may have concerns about the cancer recurring or they may need some time to feel safe. This delay is not maladaptive defensiveness. It is considered healthy adaptive coping and good use of problem-solving strategies. They remember their initial experience and distress of viewing the mastectomy. The delay may even give them a greater appreciation of the reconstruction (Schain et al.). Satisfaction is a very individual and subjective issue. Each woman must gather information and come to terms with her feelings and needs.

Choosing Not To Reconstruct

Schain (1991) states that "it's natural to wonder why a woman who has lost a breast would not choose to reconstruct." However, many women feel it is not necessary. Their life is minimally altered and it is not essential to their physical or psychological well-being. They have adopted a "pseudo-acceptance." They may feel that not having a breast is not that bad and adjust much like a woman who fails to develop at adolescence. Others may choose not to reconstruct out of a "martyr syndrome." They wear their mastectomy as a badge of courage, proof of injustice in the world, and their ability to overcome hardships (Schain et al.). Some women feel the effort is not worth it and choose to redefine their priorities and self-image. Attachment to the prosthesis may produce a reluctance to give it up. Our society remains puritanical, which may make older women inhibited and feeling as if they need permission. They may feel selfish and ungrateful, believing it is too much to expect both longevity of life and symmetry of breasts (Schain et al.).

Fears that may cause a woman not to choose reconstruction are:

- may mask reoccurrence of cancer;
- not living up to the idealized image of women's breasts;
- uncertainty of the procedure;
- fear of pain and discomfort; and
- fear of cancer reoccurrence (Schain et al.).

Strong protective feelings toward the other breast may provoke a fear that an implant may cause cancer in this surviving twin. These women may need to wait until they feel free of disease before considering reconstruction. Women 40 and over may rely on an inner sense of worth rather than physical attributes (Schain et al., 1991). Finally, the medical stage of the disease may make it physically inadvisable.

Regardless of the woman's choice to have reconstruction or to not have reconstruction, the nurse must remain supportive of the woman and her decision.

Role Of The Physician

The breast surgeon has the responsibility to discuss the possibility of breast reconstruction with his/her patient. The oncologist should communicate proposed methods of treatment of the cancer to the plastic surgeon. All physicians should work together as a team to provide the patient with optimal care. By providing information and giving approval for the patient to consult a plastic surgeon, some of the patient's fears and anxieties may be reduced. Including breast reconstruction as part of the total treatment and rehabilitation assures the patient that as much as possible will be done for her.

Pre-counseling is an important process in which accurate information is disseminated to the patient. Education of the risks, benefits and possible complications helps prepare women to make choices based on realistic possibilities. Women who anticipate a magical change in their life are often disappointed. It is essential to consider the woman's medical and psychological resources. Every woman who gets cancer and has a mastectomy should be given the choice to reconstruct.

Dealing with medical insurance companies can be time consuming and frustrating. The office manager can help by assisting with forms and making phone calls to the insurance carrier. The two words that should be avoided are cosmetic and enhancement. Insurance companies will refuse to pay for cosmetic procedures. Physicians can facilitate insurance approval by sending letters and acting as the patient's advocate. It is a wonder how any health benefit system, whether an insurance company or state medical system, could fail to recognize such a physical loss and refuse to subsidize reconstruction. Since breasts are paired organs, reconstruction should also include the contralateral breast if it is necessary to achieve symmetry.

The plastic surgical nurse begins to develop a trusting relationship with the patient upon the first visit to the office. This relationship continues and should grow in trust and confidence throughout the re-constructive process. Daily care and support should be given as well as educational information regarding procedures and outcomes.

The role of the recovery room nurse is also essential for continu-ity of care. If he/she sees the patient preoperatively, then he/she is a familiar face postoperatively. This reinforces support and trust (Matheson 8: Drever, 1990). A supportive environment allows the patient to express fears. Psychological techniques used by the nurse should focus on reducing the patient's stress and fears, such as:

- fear of death;
- fear of pain and discomfort;
- fear of anesthesia and loss of control; and
- fear of the unknown.

A moderate level of anticipatory fear is normal and considered healthy. It serves to motivate inner preparation to handle stress. The patient may become dependent on the doctor and the nurse during this time. Being available to the patient for emotional support is crucial.

Outcomes

Although most women feel positive about the results of reconstruc-tion, they also speak of some ambivalence about the repair. Expres-sions of disappointment regarding the "not-so-real" appearance of the new breast may be verbalized. They may not feel the same attach-ment to the reconstructed breast as they once had toward the real one. There may be disappointment that reconstruction did not return them to their previous state. Many women found they could not es-cape the devastating effects of breast loss and the emotional process of mourning (Kasper, 1995).

The doctor/patient relationship is critical in the patient's decision making process. If reconstruction is her hope for normalcy and the results are not satisfactory, she may take out her anger on the plas-tic surgeon. Expressions of hostility stem from a sense of helplessness and hopelessness. Despair and depression convert to anger and ani-mosity (Schain et al.). Reconstruction must not be offered as a cos-metic triumph. Yet, the more positive patient views reconstruction as restoring oneself to a sense of wholeness. Psychologically, there is a commitment to the future, an expression of the intention to live and enjoy life (Matheson & Drever, 1990).

Tram Flap Procedures

Cederna et al. (1995) found that patients reconstructed with autologous tissue were more satisfied with how the breast felt. Thirty-three patients were surveyed via telephone and a self-assessment questionnaire. Although they had more psychological, social, and physical impairments, these women reported greater satisfaction with feel and cosmetic result, with the exception of the presence of scars. There was no statistical difference in body image or overall satisfaction.

The procedure itself produced an increased level of psychological discomfort. The anticipation of a longer surgery, anesthesia, hospitalization, and physical recovery period produced greater pre-surgery anxiety. Generally, it is perceived as a more complex and deforming procedure.

Tissue Expansion Procedures

Tissue expansion is viewed as an easier, less invasive procedure. Explaining to the patient the concept of blowing up a balloon-like device to stretch and grow new skin helps prepare women for a longer course of reconstruction.

The beginning phase of tissue expansion is usually a time of excitement as the patient observes the enlarging mound. Toward the end of expansion, however, it becomes difficult to present a balanced appearance. The over-expanded breast may become uncomfortable, and the patient may become anxious, depressed or fatigued (Goin & Goin, 1988). When the expander is removed and the long-term implant is placed, the patient is usually relieved and generally pleased.

Nipple Reconstruction

Nipple reconstruction is often referred to as "finishing the job" or "the icing on the cake." There is a sense of satisfaction and wholeness that is not achieved by merely improving physical contour alone (Goin & Goin, 1988).

Conclusion

Whether a woman chooses breast reconstruction or not, a common link among breast cancer survivors is that they have faced their mortality. They have a depth of emotion that can be heard in their voices, seen in their eyes, and felt through their hearts.

The concerns, fears, and emotions of these patients echo a triumph over cancer and sometimes even death. To them, life has become a precious gift. Their spirit, courage, and honesty are an inspiration to us all.

References/Readings

Bartelink, H., Van Dam, F., & Van Dongen, J. (1985). Psychological effects of breast conserving therapy In comparison with radical mastectomy. *Radiation Oncology*, 11(2),381-385.

Cederna, P.S., Yates, W.R., Chang, P., & Cram, A.E., & Ricciardelli, E.J. (1995). Postmastectomy reconstruction: Comparative analysis of the psychosocial, functional, and cosmetic effects of transverse rectus abdominis musculocutaneous flap versus breast implant reconstruction. *Annals of Plastic Surgery*, 35(5) 458-468.

Clifford, E., Clifford, M., & Georgiade, N.G. (1984). The meaning of concepts related to breast reconstruction. *Annals of Plastic Surgery*, 13(1), 34-37.

Corsten, L.A., Suduikis S.V, & Donegan W.L. (1992). Patient satisfaction with breast reconstruction. *Wisconsin Medical Journal*, 125-129.

Foster, J.B., McKenney, S.A., Hayes, D.F., Bushnell, S.S., Card, I.C., Quadrino, A., & Griesemer, S. (1991). Psychosocial issues in breast reconstruction. *Cancer*, 68(5), 1176-1177.

Franchelli, S., Leone, M.S., Berrino, P., Passarelli, B., Capelli, M., Baracco, G., Alberisio, A., Morasso, G., & Santi, P.L. (1995). Psychological evaluation of patients undergoing breast reconstruction using two different methods: Autologous tissues versus prostheses. *Plastic and Reconstructive Surgery*, 95(7), 1213-1220.

Goin, M.K., & Goin, J.M. (1988). Growing pains: The psychological experience of breast reconstruction with tissue expansion. *Annals of Plastic Surgery*, 21(3), 217-222.

Goldberg, R, Stolzman, M.A., & Goldberg, H.M. (1984). Psychological considerations in breast reconstruction. *Annals of Plastic Surgery*, 13(1), 3843.

Jones, D.N., & Reznikoff, M. (1989). Psychosocial adjustment to a mastectomy. *The Journal of Nervous and Mental Disease*, 177(10), 624-631.

Kasper, A.S. (1995). The social construction of breast loss and reconstruction. *Women's Health*, pages 197-219.

Kiebert, G.M., de Haes, J.C.J.M., & van De Velde, C.J.H. (1991). The impact of breast-conserving treatment and mastectomy on the quality of life of early-stage breast cancer patients: A review. *Journal of Clinical Oncology*, 9(6), 1059-1070.

Lasry, J.M., Margolese, R.G., Poisson, R., Shibata, H. Fleischer, D., Lafleur, D., Legault, S., & Taillefer, S. (1987). Depression and body image following mastectomy and lumpectomy. *Journal of Chronic Dieases*, 40(6), 529-534.

Matheson, G., & Drever, J.M. (1990). Psychological preparation of the patient for breast reconstruction. *Annals of Plastic Surgery*, 24(3), 238-247.

Rowland, J.H., Holland, J.C., Chaglassian, T, & Kinne, D. (1993). Psychological response to breast reconstruction. *Psychosomatics*, 34(3), 241-250.

Schain, W.S., Jacobs, E., & Wellisch, D.K. Psychosocial issues in breast reconstruction. *Symposium on Advances in Breast Reconstruction*, pages 237251.

Schain, W.S. (1991, September 1). Breast reconstruction. *Cancer*, supplement, pages 1170-1175.

Schain, W.S., Wellisch, D.K., Pasnau, R.O., & Landsverk, J. (1985). The sooner the better: A study of psychological factors in women undergoing immediate versus delayed breast reconstruction. *American Journal of Psychiatry*, 142(1), 4046.

Vinokur, A.D., Threatt, B.A., Vinodur-Kaplan, D., & Satariano, W.A. (1990). The process of recovery from breast cancer for younger and older patients. *Cancer*, 65, 1242-1253.

Wellisch, D.K., Schain, W.S., Noone, R.B., & Little, J.W, III (1987). The psychological contribution of nipple addition in breast reconstruction. *Plastic and Reconstructive Surgery*, 80(5), 699-704.

Diane Hart, RN, is the Patient Coordinator for MENTOR H/S in Santa Barbara, CA. She has been a surgical nurse for 26 years, and has specialized in plastic and reconstructive surgery for eight of those years.

Chapter 48

Taking Five: Braving High-Risk Surgery, Matthew Scott Receives a Transplanted Hand

Dawn Scott bends to kiss her husband, Matt, as he sits in a chair at Louisville, Kentucky's Jewish Hospital. "He has such a beautiful face," she says lovingly. He doesn't contradict her—though to be fair, he is preoccupied with another part of his anatomy: his heavily bandaged left hand. "It's amazing," says Scott, 37, whose left arm, for the first time in 13 years, doesn't end at the wrist. After undergoing the nation's first hand transplant, the onetime paramedic from Absecon, N.J., who had his dominant hand blown off by a firecracker in 1985, is gazing on fingertips that only days before belonged to a brain-dead stranger.

If all goes well, Scott will be able to pick up most objects and perhaps even button his shirt or tie his shoes, which he can't do easily with the prosthesis. And aside from the psychological boost, he should have some sense of touch. "This is just a fledgling attempt," admits Dr. Warren Breidenbach, 52, head of the 17-member surgical team that performed the 14 1/2-hour procedure. In fact, the world's first known try at a hand transplant took place in Ecuador in 1964, but after two weeks the recipient's body rejected it. No other attempts were made until last September, when New Zealander Clint Hallam received a hand in Lyons, France, so far without major complications.

"If we can make transplantation of the hand viable," says Breidenbach, "we can do the breast, face, jaw, knee, or elbow." If Scott's transplant provides new hope for the maimed, it is also a little eerie: wearing an outward part of another person—not a hidden heart or kidney, but the instrument of gesture, caress and even, through fingerprints, identity. But above all, the transplant is a gamble. The odds are 30 to 50 percent that Scott's immune system will reject the transplant in the first year. And even if he clears that hurdle, he must spend the rest of his life on immunosuppressive drugs, leaving him open to any number of life-threatening infections and illnesses. Moreover, Scott has diabetes, which the drugs make more difficult to control.

Some in the medical community question the wisdom of endangering his life for what they call a cosmetic measure. "It's definitely experimental surgery with high risks," says Dr. Bill Cooney of the Mayo Clinic, president-elect of the American Society for Surgery of the Hand. "We just pray that this young man has a successful outcome—by success, I mean survival." Arthur Caplan, director of the University of Pennsylvania's Center for Bioethics, wonders if the surgery should have been reserved for a double amputee. "If one hand is missing, most people do okay with a prosthesis," he says. "[In this case] telling someone he might be dead in seven or eight years from the drugs is a little harder to justify." Scott, whose wife is a nurse and who is himself a supervisor for a New Jersey health-care company, understood the risks. But though his battery-powered prosthesis allowed him to work, to him that wasn't the point. "No matter how good they make the prosthesis, it is not real," he says. "It is not flesh and blood and bone, and that's what I want back." Dawn, 34, frets about complications—and the possibility of rejection. "It would be almost like losing his hand all over again," she says. "That would be more devastating in a lot of ways."

The first time was traumatic enough. After a night of partying on Dec. 23, 1985, Scott went to a friend's house, where he found an M-80 firecracker. After lighting it with his cigarette, he started to carry it outside when it went off in his hand. "I saw the devastation and the blood," he says. "Immediately I believed the life I'd known was over." The hand was beyond saving, so Scott agreed to amputation. Recuperating at the home of his mother, Mary Lou, he suffered phantom pains, but even worse was the anguish. "I had all those feelings of rage and depression," he says. The handless arm was "a constant, something I looked at every day and hated."

After three months he was sufficiently healed to wear the prosthesis, which opens and closes when forearm muscles are flexed. "I had to learn how much pressure to apply when I pick something up," says Scott. He practiced on eggs, breaking dozens before he got it right. Scott went back to work, starting as a dispatcher, then returned to the field. (His scariest challenge was the first time he delivered a baby with one hand. "I was absolutely sure I was going to drop that kid," he says.) He met Dawn in 1986; they married in 1992 and have two sons, Ian, 7, and Jeremy, 2. They were vacationing in London when Dawn read of the Louisville surgeons' plans to attempt the country's first hand transplant.

The next day Matt called and was granted an interview—along with some caveats. "We asked Matt, 'What if you die?'" says Breidenbach. "He understood what we were talking about." Scott was then placed on a waiting list for a donor hand of compatible size, bone structure, skin tone, and blood type.

The call came at 2 a.m. on Jan. 24; by 11:30 the Scotts had flown from Philadelphia to Louisville, and Matt was being prepped for surgery. The donor's heart was still beating when surgeons removed the hand, which was brought in a cooler to Jewish Hospital. At 3:36 p.m. the operation began. Screws and titanium plates were used to attach the bone, then Breidenbach hooked up the blood vessels. Thirteen years had passed since they had carried blood to a hand, and there was no guarantee they would work. "Vessels don't do well when you ask them all of a sudden to start spitting out blood," Breidenbach explains. "And you don't have anything if the blood doesn't flow." The surgeons were elated as Scott's newly attached hand flushed pink. When Scott's atrophied tendons proved too short to support the hand, microsurgeon Tsu-Min Tsai supplemented them with tendons from the feet. "If you are in trouble, you call Dr. Tsai," says Breidenbach. "He's a human sewing machine."

As of early this month, Scott could flex his wrist and curl his fingers, and though it may be a year before he has feeling in the hand, his circulation is excellent. Ahead lie months of therapy and a life clouded by uncertainty but so far not by regret. "This is a risk I need to take," Scott says simply, "because it is what I want."

—by Richard Jerome and Giovanna Breu

Chapter 49

The Story of Replantation and Microsurgery

Very few surgical achievements underline the importance of a team effort as much as the first attempt at successful surgical replantation. This event took place in Boston's Massachusetts General Hospital on May 21, 1962. Dr. Ronald Malt, a general surgical resident, had been dispatched in the Massachusetts General Hospital ambulance that day and brought in an injured boy whose right arm was severed below the shoulder. Malt brought the amputated arm with the patient and then persuaded a group of surgeons from several specialties to attempt to 'replant' the limb. The development of replantation began that late afternoon as the team of surgeons determined to salvage the amputated arm by shortening and stabilizing the two fragments of the humerus, anastomosing the severed arteries and veins, stitching the four severed nerves and repairing the cut bulk of muscles.

This first successful replantation of an amputated upper extremity started a cascade of stimulating responses in many areas and in different countries. In reply to my inquiry regarding what thoughts had stirred in his mind during that momentous event, Malt wrote that he had no preconceived idea of replanting the limb. The immediate

"The Story of Replantation and Microsurgery, Including the Contribution of Canadian Surgeons," Martin A. Entin MD, CM, MSc, FRCSC, FACS, Royal Victoria Hospital, Montreal, Quebec, from *The Canadian Journal of Plastic Surgery,* vol. 5., no. 4, Winter 1997. © 1997, The Canadian Journal of Plastic Surgery; reprinted with permission.

challenge of persuading several specialists to participate in a 'wonderful experiment' produced general agreement, and the individual contributions merged into an unprecedented team effort.

This successful replantation would not have been possible without the preliminary development of microsurgical techniques during the late 1950s. J.H. Jacobson and his associates had established that an operating microscope is indispensable for success with anastomosing vessels of less than 2 mm in diameter. The gentle handling of small vessels and the use of miniature delicate instruments then became common practice, and many surgeons have attempted to work with small vessels during their experimental laboratory training. Repair of severed digital vessels in the early 1960s was carried out with a 50 percent success rate.

Malt's replantation of an amputated upper extremity was largely a synthesis of existing skills and knowledge. "I hate to think what might have happened if we had bungled," wrote Malt in June 1995 (personal communication). Within one year of the successful replantation, Chinese surgeons began their own series of replantation of forearms, hands and digits; within 10 years they startled the Western world with their successes. China was in the midst of industrial development during the 1960s, but the machines that they used were primitive and without sufficient safety devices. It was not surprising that China had the world's near monopoly of amputations. Chairman Mao gave the project of 'salvaging our workers' hands' the first priority. While the Western world rested on the glory of the first successful arm replantation, there was less success with digital replantation because of a lack of appropriate small instruments, sutures and skill.

Inspired by Glaswegian plastic surgeon Thomas Gibson in 1957, the young American surgeon, Harry Buncke, pioneered the development of the new specialty of microsurgery. Handling of very small vessels required the creation of 'micro-instruments' efficient in handling the delicate structures. The greatest obstacle was producing a small thread with an appropriate surgical needle that would permit sewing the walls of the blood vessels without excessive injury.

Buncke showed great ingenuity by using a method of depositing microscopic metallic ions directly onto the thread, giving it a needle-like stiffness. Despite his assiduous effort, it took Buncke seven years to achieve successful replantation of an amputated rabbit ear involving vessels about 1 mm in external diameter. In 1965, he successfully replanted the amputated index and thumb of a Rhesus monkey. Buncke's pioneering efforts were reported in some detail, underlining the fact that this new field demanded dedication and ingenuity in developing special instruments, as well as perseverance in acquiring high skill. In July 1965, S. Tamai replanted a human thumb; John Cobbett of East Grinstead completed the first great toe-to-thumb transfer in 1968. Buncke achieved great toe-to-thumb transplant in 1972 (personal communication). Small vessel anastomosis had become practical.

Chinese Experience

Reports of dramatic successes in replantation by Chinese surgeons were published in 1965. The reports of successful replantations of 'scores' of amputated arms and 'hundreds' of digits challenged the belief of Western surgeons. There had been little contact with China during the preceding decade, and consequently Chinese surgeons' amazing achievements remained as hearsay until verified.

However, the Chinese reports stirred up great interest among North American replantation surgeons, who organized the North American Replantation Mission (ARM) and were finally permitted to visit China to examine the large number of successful replantations in several Chinese surgical centers. The importance of this intellectual, academic, technical and surgical exchange, preceded by a period of virtual isolation, was beneficial to both Chinese surgeons and members of ARM. The Chinese surgeons were quick to follow-up on Malt's procedure of successful replantation of upper limbs and proceeded to develop their own technique utilizing primitive instruments and only small magnifying loops (instead of operating microscopes). They achieved an overall success rate of 50 percent to 60 percent.

Dr. Ch'en Chung Wei, the Chief of Orthopaedic Service of the Sixth People's Hospital in Shanghai, China, was encouraged by Chairman Mao to establish a special center for the replantation of amputated parts. Dr. Ch'en shared his experience with the members of ARM during our visit to China in 1973. While he was given 'an official carte blanche' to restore 'the workers' hands', Ch'en was unsatisfied with the initial results of the replantation of amputated digits. The final result of only 50 percent to 60 percent success was frustrating; he did not understand the physiopathological process that prevented achievement of total success.

As he described it, and as every replantation surgeon had observed, the frustrations were as follows: as soon as the artery of the replanted digit is connected by anastomosis and the clamps are removed, the amputated portion of the digit flushes with the inflow of the blood. Usually, the vein is repaired at this time and subsequently the repair of the nerve is carried out. In most of the cases, the finger will remain pink throughout the period of healing. In some replants a dusky color appears at the tip of the finger within 24 hour, which may increase over the next few days, suggesting that the stagnation of circulation has taken place. The color of the finger may become darker, and gangrene may set in with loss of the replant. Most of us are only too familiar with this process.

Ch'en told us that he observed this sequence of events in 19 consecutive digital implants. Realizing that there was something wrong in what he was doing, Ch'en retreated for a couple of weeks into a commune to attempt to solve this problem. The traditional Chinese retreat consisted of working hard by day and reading Chairman Mao's Red Book by night.

Ch'en found that the physical exertion of life in the commune left little desire to read Mao's book. After a period of adjustment, however, he was able to read a few pages. One evening while reading a certain section of the Red Book, Ch'en was startled to come across a passage that seemed to have a direct bearing on the problem that frustrated him. The passage read: "In dealing with forces of unequal strength, one has to strengthen the weak to overcome the strong."

In recounting this story to the members of ARM Ch'en said "What a simple solution!" Noticing the puzzled expression on the faces of the Western guests, Ch'en explained that in replantation, the surgeon deals with two forces: one is strong, the dynamic arterial circulation, and the other is weak, the passive venous circulation. Mao's passage suggested to Ch'en that it was the weak venous circulation that was the problem. To correct this, one had to strengthen this weak element.

The solution was clear to Ch'en. The loss of a finger occurred despite the initial arterial inflow. It was the inadequacy of venous drainage that created a gradual increasing passive hyperemia with venous stagnation and led to the death of the tissue. Most surgeons traditionally connected one artery and one vein. Mao's admonition, however, suggested reinforcing the weak to overcome the strong.

Ch'en could not wait to get to the hospital to try connecting two or three veins for each digit, which solved the problem of inadequate venous Drainage. Mao's advice, in fact, led to the eventual improvement of all replantations. Afterwards Chinese surgeons achieved 80 percent survival of reimplanted complete amputations (Figures 49.1. and 49.2.). Sixty percent of such patients returned to their original work, and 20 percent had to change to less demanding jobs. Moreover, they achieved the successful transplant of the left foot to replace the crushed right foot in a patient with bilateral amputation of both legs (Figure 49.3.).

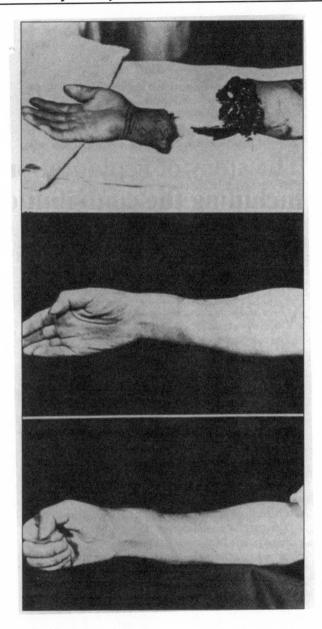

Figure 49.1. *Photographs of a 37-year-old male patient who was shown to the North American Replantation Mission (ARM) during the visit to Peking Hospital. The original injury occurred in 1964 (top). Examination nine years after injury (in 1973) showed normal sensation and good range of motion (middle and bottom).*

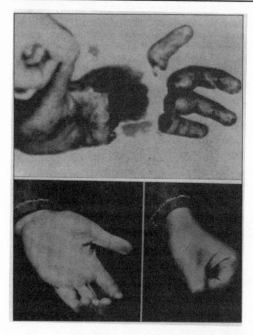

Figure 49.2. A female worker shown to the North American Replantation Mission in No. 6 People's Hospital of Shanghai seven years after replantation of three of the four amputated fingers (top). When we saw her in 1973 (bottom left and right), she was able to knit and play the accordion.

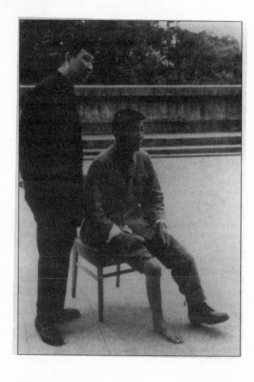

Figure 49.3. A male patient seen by the North American Replantation Mission (ARM) in Hangchow was the first successful cross-foot replantation in a bilateral amputation. His right foot was badly crushed. The undamaged left foot of the below-knee amputation was replanted to replace the right foot. ARM saw the patient in 1973, two years after replantation.

The discussion among the members of ARM and the Chinese surgeons that took place at the various cities we visited outlined the areas that needed further work. We left an operating microscope for the surgeons of the Sixth People's Hospital in Shanghai. The symbiosis that resulted from the exchange of valuable information with the Chinese was beneficial to both sides. Dr. Ch'en was invited by the author to present his findings at the Microsurgical Symposium at McGill University in January 1974 and at the Annual Meeting of the American Society for Surgery of the Hand, which was held in Dallas a few weeks later.

Canadian Contribution to Microsurgery and Replantation

McGill University

Dr. Bruce Williams of McGill University had a sustained interest in microvascular anastomosis. He attempted to transplant a rabbit ear by maintaining microcirculation with the use of a miniature artificial respirator. While the transplanted ear could be preserved for a few days, it did not survive. It was obvious that the direct anastomosis of vessels still had to be achieved.

In developing the technique for anastomosis of small blood vessels at the Montreal General Hospital, Dr. Williams found direct suturing with the aid of the microscope to be more efficient than using a mechanical stapler to repair small vessels. The experimental nerve repair using the microscope was carried out by Julie Terzis, Michael Orgel and Burt Faibisoff under Dr. Williams' supervision. In 1972, at an International Seminar on Sutures, Dr. Williams raised the possibility of transferring tissue flaps with no blood supply by immediate microvascular anastomosis.

In 1973, Dr. Rolland K. Daniel participated with Dr. Williams in research related to free transfers of flaps by the direct suture of arteries and veins using a microsurgical technique. They achieved a successful free flap transfer in the pig. Later that year Daniel obtained further training in Australia. In collaboration with Mr. Ian Taylor, the Australian plastic surgeon, he performed the first free flap transfer in a human. The procedure involved the transfer of a free flap from the groin to a large defect on the denuded ankle of Taylor's patient.

Following the Microsurgical Symposium at McGill in 1974, several successful replantations of amputated digits took place at McGill University. The experimental work kept expanding to involve the study of free muscle transplants. This experiment was carried out by Dr. J.K. Terzis of McGill and Dalhousie University of Halifax in association with Drs. Williams and R.W. Dykes. The research subsequently extended to the microvascular transfer of ribs and scapular bone grafts involving several research fellows under the general supervision of Dr. Williams.

Before the free transfer of tissue by vascular anastomosis, the transfer of tissues was cumbersome, time-consuming and often uncomfortable to the patient. Even a transfer by means of pedicle required 'delays' to ensure adequate circulation. For example, the frequently used cross-leg flap, which provided skin cover from one leg to a defect on the other, often required complicated immobilization with a plaster cast for several weeks.

The development of microsurgical skill, which permitted the replantation of limbs and digits, enabled plastic surgeons to transplant successfully a free skin flap, parts of muscles, bones, and compound skin and bone. This rapid transplant of various tissues resulted in a great savings of hospital time and discomfort to the patient.

Whole joint transplantation: The author has carried out a series of transplantation joints in rats, dogs and humans. The findings show that while joints with reconstituted vascular supply survived, they showed the degenerative changes similar to denervated Charcot joints. Whole-joint transplants with preserved neurovascular bundles in dogs retain all criteria of full viability and function. Similar findings had been found in the transplantation of joints in rats and Rhesus monkeys carried out by Buncke and his associates when blood and nerve supply were reestablished. It appears that the vascular element is necessary for the immediate survival of the joint. The nerve supply is needed to prevent the degenerative changes associated with the continuous stress of function. In replanted digits in humans containing one or two joints, normal function was restored if normal nerve function was re-established.

Neurovascular free flap: It was essential that the distribution of the vascular component corresponded precisely with the sensory one in a neurovascular free flap in order to give the greatest sensory function when the flap was applied to an anesthetic area. While the vascular distribution could be ascertained by direct inspection and/ or by applying the Doppler effect, it was impossible to predict the sensory distribution. Dr. Julia Terzis devised an ingenious method of determining the sensory distribution in the skin. Dr. Ramon Y. Cajal described the new method as follows: when the small hairs in the skin are deflected, the afferent fibers associated with the hair produce an electrical stimulation; this electrical current is very small, but can be magnified in intensity so that it becomes possible to trace its distribution into the network of sensory nerves. In 1974, Terzis and her associates were able to achieve sensory mapping of skin flaps using this technique. This method permitted an accurate assessment of sensory distribution of neurovascular donor flaps for anesthetic areas.

University of Toronto Contribution

Dr. Nancy McKee established a microsurgical laboratory at the University of Toronto Medical Science Building with which Ralph Manktelow was associated for several years. Dr. W.K. Lindsay, Chairman of the University of Toronto Division of Plastic Surgery, helped to form the Plastic Surgery Replantation Team so that coverage by skilful personnel was available in the participating hospitals. Lindsay felt that only surgeons who had acquired fine microsurgical skills should be chosen for that team, which comprised Dr. Ralph Manktelow from Toronto General Hospital; Drs. Jim Mahoney and Nancy McKee from St Michael's Hospital; and Dr. Ron Zucker from The Hospital for Sick Children.

In his personal reminiscences about the early development of replantation, Lindsay, now Professor Emeritus, recalled that replantation had received considerable stimulus in Toronto in 1974 during the visit by the delegation of Chinese surgeons. They were especially impressed by the Chinese results of replantation presented by the delegation's leader, Ch'en Chung Wei (personal communication).

The University of Toronto Replantation Team was very active in the 1970s. Fifty-two patients were operated on at the Toronto General Hospital from 1974 to 1979 by Manktelow and McKee. In 1979, they analyzed the results of 20 patients from that group who were followed for more than 2.5 years. The series comprised 33 replanted digits with an 85-percent rate of survival. The average two-point discrimination was 8 mm; eight of the 12 compensation workers in that group returned to their original work (66 percent). Sensitivity to cold was a persistent complication in a large portion of the patients.

Based on their analysis of these 20 patients, Manktelow and McKee made the following recommendations: replantation of one or two amputated fingers is not worthwhile; replantation of the fingers at the transmetacarpal level is desirable; and replantation is questionable in extensive crushing injuries.

University of Saskatoon

A very interesting account of the development of replantation and microsurgery at the University of Saskatchewan comes from the detailed reminiscences of Dr. C. Vaughan A. Bowen. He trained as an orthopedic surgeon but later acquired skills in replantation at the Vancouver General Hospital and with Mr. Bernard O'Brien in Melbourne, Australia. He was invited to start a replantation service in the University of Saskatchewan in 1983 and developed an active liaison with the plastic surgery service there. The first patient who underwent a vascularization had an ischemic thumb, and the patient did well. The first replantation was done on a farmer who had amputated his thumb through the proximal phalanx.

Dr. Bowen assembled a team of microvascular surgeons in Saskatoon: Drs. Ron Miliken, Geoff Johnston and Brian Clapson. This team replanted a large number of digits and avulsion amputations of the thumb. With the help of the University Hospital Foundation grant in 1985, Dr. Bowen set up a microsurgical laboratory, which served to train residents in orthopedic and plastic surgery.

Criteria for Assessment of Sensory Recovery after Replantation

It is obvious that the two most critical components in replantation are the blood vessels (arteries and veins) and nerves. If the blood supply to the replant is not immediately successful, or cannot be quickly restored, the replanted unit dies. The regeneration of the repaired nerves, however, is a gradual process, extending over many months. Poor recovery of the sensory element interferes with the function of the replant and may produce undesirable sequelae, such as hypersensitivity and intolerance to cold.

The reproducible assessment of functional recovery after nerve injury is especially difficult. Dr. Erik Moberg was the first to offer tangible reproducible measurements for sensory recovery. He used the ninhydrin test and two-point discrimination to measure the progressive recovery after nerve repair. Moberg also devised a procedure to measure the tactile gnosis and stereognosis, the capacity to recognize standard small objects, as the final assessment of sensory recovery. These findings were reproduced and became adapted as criteria for the assessment of sensory recovery or nerve injury after transplantation.

In a remarkable study reported by L.T. Glickman and S. MacKinnon, sensory recovery following the replantation of digits was compared with that of a large series of nerve repairs and nerve grafts. They found that replanted fingers regained only 50 percent of recovery, and replanted thumbs 60 percent, as measured by two-point discrimination. They noted that the recovery was considerably better in younger patients, and recommended sensory education during the recovery period to improve the final results of replantation.

Summary

While the early development of replantation was an international effort, in time Canadian researchers and surgeons made important contributions to the field. Moreover, Canadians contributed significantly to the evolution of transplantation of free skin pedicles, bones and other tissues. Canadian surgeons have also made a notable contribution to the development of microsurgery.

This review of replantation benefited from the personal reminiscences of North American replantation surgeons. Reports of some of the Canadian centers did not arrive in time for publication. I would like to express my appreciation to all participants.

Correspondence and reprints: Dr. Martin A. Entin, Royal Victoria Hospital, 687 Pine Avenue West, Montreal, Quebec H3A 1A1. Telephone: 514-843-1231, fax: 514-843-1468.

Acknowledgements: The McGill Institute of the Study of Canada supported part of this project.

Chapter 50

Gender Reassignment Surgical Procedures

Contents

Section 50.1

Vaginoplasty

Gender Reassignment Surgery (GRS) in Montreal from their web site at
http://www.grsmontreal.com. © 2000; reprinted with permission.

Gender Reassignment Surgery (GRS) in Montreal performs the
"skin inversion technique" for vaginoplasty. Dr. Ménard's refinements
of the skin inversion technique have redefined the standards of vaginoplasty and are responsible for the most enviable reputation of
Montreal as one of the world's best centers for GRS. Cosmetic and
functional results are outstanding and state-of-the-art: skin hooding
(prepuce) over the clitoris, excellent vaginal depth, vaginal opening
with labia minora and without late contractures (posterior band).

Skin Inversion Technique

After surgery, our caring and experienced personnel will show you
how to achieve dilation and proper hygiene. For this purpose, you will
be given your own molds and bidet which you will carry back home.
The vaginoplasty is a two and a half hour procedure under general
anesthesia. If desired, breast augmentation and/or Adam's apple shaving can be combined with your vaginoplasty. If you are considering
vaginoplasty, GRS provides a complete information package: color
brochure (with pictures of possible results), personal medical history
documents, criteria of eligibility and specific information on preparation before surgery, surgical technique,and dilation program.

For more information contact: Clinique de chirurgie esthétique St-
Joseph, 1003, boul. St-Joseph Est, Montréal (Québec), H2J 1L2., (514)
288-2097; Fax: (514) 288-3547; e-mail: info@grsmontreal.com.

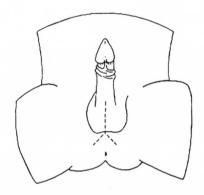

Figure 50.1. *Skin incisions on the penis shaft and perineum.*

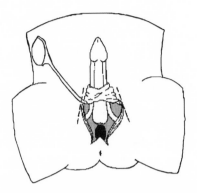

Figure 50.2. *Removal of testicles and penis skin degloving.*

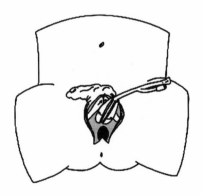

Figure 50.3. *Penis is amputated, mucosal flap for the clitoris, vaginal cavity is opened.*

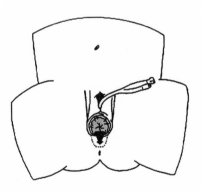

Figure 50.4. *Skin inverted with mold inside the cavity, skin hooding (prepuce) over the clitoris.*

Section 50.2

Adam's Apple Shaving

Gender Reassignment Surgery in Montreal from their web site at http://www.grsmontreal.com. © 2000; reprinted with permission.

Adam's apple shaving or "chondrolaryngoplasty" is aimed at correcting an unpleasing bulge at the anterior neck. (Figure 50.5) This minor procedure can be done under local anesthesia through a convenient skin crease and leaves a short, horizontal and concealable scar at the anterior neck. If desired, it can be combined with vaginoplasty and/or breast augmentation under general anesthesia.

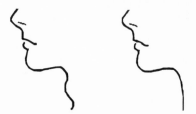

Figure 50.5. *Adam's Apple Shaving*

In the long term, it will not modify adversely your voice tonality and the unwanted "apple" will not grow back. In a short operative time, between 30 and 45 minutes, you can get rid of a constant embarrassment and your neck will fit your individual gender.

For more information contact: Clinique de chirurgie esthétique St-Joseph, 1003, boul. St-Joseph Est, Montréal (Québec), H2J 1L2., (514) 288-2097; Fax: (514) 288-3547; e-mail: info@grsmontreal.com.

Section 50.3

Voice Surgery

Gender Reassignment Surgery (GRS) in Montreal from their web site at
www.grsmontreal.com. © 2000; reprinted with permission.

The fundamental frequency or pitch is the quality of voice that can
be modified with surgery. Vocal register, intensity and vocal tract resonance (e.g., vowel production) also can be changed, but only with
speech therapy.

The mechanical properties of the vocal cords have to be altered to
modify pitch. This can be done directly by scarring procedures on the
cords (laser and cauterization), but they are unpredictable, irreversible and often need revisions. On the other hand, it can be done safely
by indirect cricothyroid approximation.

Cricothyroid approximation increases the tension in the vocal cords
and consequently raises the frequency from a male pattern (100-150
Hz) to a female one (200-300 Hz). Preferably, the procedure is done
under local anesthesia through a short neck incision and can be combined with Adam's apple shaving if desired. It requires a short operation time (one hour) during which you will notice an immediate

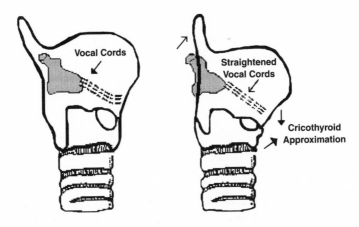

Figure 50.6. *Before and after cricothyroid approximation.*

299

change. Voice rest is recommended after surgery for a short period and the final result comes gradually within the first six to 12 months. Speech therapy is advised before and after surgery.

For more information contact: Clinique de chirurgie esthétique St-Joseph, 1003, boul. St-Joseph Est, Montréal (Québec), H2J 1L2., (514) 288-2097; Fax: (514) 288-3547; e-mail: info@grsmontreal.com.

Section 50.4

Breast Augmentation

Gender Reassignment Surgery (GRS) in Montreal from their web site at www.grsmontreal.com. © 2000; reprinted with permission.

Breast augmentation is often requested to enforces one's perception of feminine gender and give a well proportioned figure. It is performed, most of the time, in combination with another procedure. For example, breast augmentation can be combined with vaginoplasty

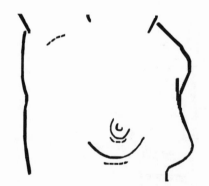

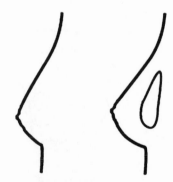

Figure 50.7. Breast augmentation incisions (only one per breast is necessary).

Figure 50.8. Insertion of the breast implant increases breast volume.

and/or Adam's apple shaving and/or rhinoplasty. It adds approximately 60 minutes to the operating time and needless to say, in can be done as a separate procedure.

To achieve chest fullness, saline-filled implants are inserted under your existing breast. Being used since the 70s, they have a long history of safety and their reliability has increased to a very acceptable level. Other implants could be available in the near future, pending strong scientific data for their use.

The location of the incisions, volume of augmentation, location of implants (either subglandular or submuscular) are some of the important points that have to be discussed with your surgeon, who will take into account your particular needs and goals, individual features and anatomy.

For more information contact: Clinique de chirurgie esthétique St-Joseph, 1003, boul. St-Joseph Est, Montréal (Québec), H2J 1L2., (514) 288-2097; Fax: (514) 288-3547; e-mail: info@grsmontreal.com.

Section 50.5

Phalloplasty

Gender Reassignment Surgery (GRS) in Montreal from their web site at
www.grsmontreal.com. © 2000; reprinted with permission.

A phalloplasty is the construction of male external genitalia (phallus). You will be best served by free forearm flap phalloplasty if you seek the following objectives: genitalia that allows one to urinate while standing, a phallus with erogenous and protective sensation that grants intercourse, and pleasing aesthetics. With phalloplasty, your female genitals will be transformed to the male counterpart. There will not be any appearing female genitals. With microscopic techniques, we are performing this state-of-the-art surgery and you will

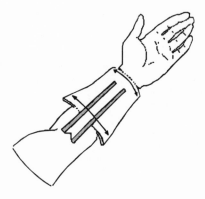

Figure 50.9. Forearm skin is elevated.

Figure 50.10. Construction of the penis around a catheter.

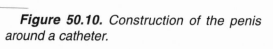

be surprised to know that it is most probably within your financial capabilities.

Male sexual organs are constructed in a two-stage procedure. The first stage is a five- to six-hour procedure done by two surgical teams.

Free-Flap Phalloplasty

Your non-dominant forearm skin, along with its sensory nerves, veins and arteries, is taken to construct the urethra, glans and penis shaft. The vaginal cavity is obstructed, the labia majora are used to construct the scrotum. The nerves responsible for clitoris sensation are preserved and after being connected, they will grow gradually into your new penis. We have not yet seen one patient who lost his capacity for orgasms after phalloplasty.

Attachment of the penis is done by connecting the two urethras, clitoris nerves to the new penis nerves and the artery and veins to the groin area. One suprapubic catheter is used to empty the bladder and another one for the urethra during healing. Your stay at the hospital will last a week, after which you will spend two more weeks at the Residence.

When protective sensation of the penis has recovered, approximately six to nine months after the first stage, testicular implants and implants to obtain rigidity (erection) on demand are inserted. For now, we use the implants available on the market that were designed for impotence. being involved in biomaterial research, we expect to release a phalloplasty designed implant in the next three or four years.

For more information contact: Clinique de chirurgie esthétique St-Joseph, 1003, boul. St-Joseph Est, Montréal (Québec), H2J 1L2., (514) 288-2097; Fax: (514) 288-3547; e-mail: info@grsmontreal.com.

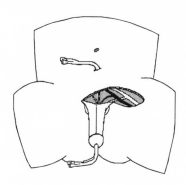

Figure 50.11. *Penis is connected in its proper location.*

Section 50.6

Clitoris Sparing Procedures

Gender Reassignment Surgery (GRS) in Montreal from their web site at
www.grsmontreal.com. © 2000; reprinted with permission.

You may want to preserve some of your female genitals or you may
not want to undergo a complete free-flap phalloplasty. Then you have
two possibilities: metaidoioplasty or locoregional flaps.

Metaidoioplasty consists of the transformation of your female
external genitals into the male counterpart. The technique releases
your actual clitoris to get it somewhat longer, uses the labia minora
to form the urethra inside the penis, moves the your labia majora to
form the scrotum, and testicular implants can be inserted inside.
Metaidoioplasty will not allow intercourse and will appear as if you
"just had a cold shower." It is a suitable alternative if testosterone
(male hormones) enlarged significantly your clitoris and if you already
have a satisfactory sexual life. With this procedure, you can elect to
get your vaginal cavity closed and/or urethra connected.

Locoregional flaps from the groin and abdomen have been used
for many years and are the predecessors of the state-of-the-art free-
flap phalloplasty. They allow only phallic volume and length. Sensation is not possible and it is a lengthy process (multi-stage). GRS
Montreal does not perform these flaps because they offer less-than-
optimal results, and in our opinion, do not fulfill the basic goals and
needs of gender reassignment surgery. However, we are ready to help
anyone with an incomplete or unfavorable result from a previous
phalloplasty.

For more information contact: Clinique de chirurgie esthétique St-
Joseph, 1003, boul. St-Joseph Est, Montréal (Québec), H2J 1L2., (514)
288-2097; Fax: (514) 288-3547; e-mail: info@grsmontreal.com.

Section 50.7

Subcutaneous Mastectomy

Gender Reassignment Surgery (GRS) in Montreal from their web site at
www.grsmontreal.com. © 2000; reprinted with permission.

Subcutaneous mastectomy is the reduction of breast volume to that
of a male-appearing chest. It is usually done alone but can be combined with a metaidoioplasty or hysterectomy and ovariectomy (neither of which are yet available at GRS Montreal). It is performed
through a semicircular "U-shaped" incision located at the junction of
normal skin and areolar skin. The incision leaves minimal scarring.

Liposuction can be used to help during the procedure in necessary,
but alone it can never remove enough breast tissue to achieve optimal results.

Subcutaneous mastectomy never needs to be done through long
transverse and conventional mastectomy or mastopexy incisions. Even
if there is significant skin laxity or excess, we still use a minimal incision (U-shaped) at the junction of the areola with the skin. After

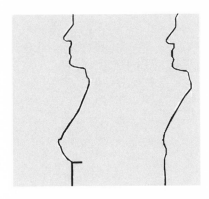

Figure 50.12. *Before and after subcutaneous mastectomy.*

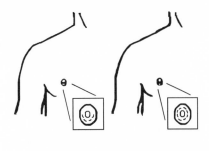

Figure 50.13. *Scar location on the chest after subcutaneous mastectomy without (left and with (right) skin laxity removal.*

surgery, natural skin retraction occurs and can correct the residual skin laxity. If it persists after a few months, we prefer to correct the remaining problem under local anesthesia. In this way you will get the least scarring, most probably a circular scar around the areola.

For more information contact: Clinique de chirurgie esthétique St-Joseph, 1003, boul. St-Joseph Est, Montréal (Québec), H2J 1L2., (514) 288-2097; Fax: (514) 288-3547; e-mail: info@grsmontreal.com.

Part Five

Additional Help and Information

Chapter 51

Glossary of Terms Used in Plastic Surgery

A

Abdominoplasty (or "tummy tuck"): a surgical procedure to remove excess fat and skin from the abdomen resulting in a flatter abdomen.

Apert's Syndrome: a rare birth defect that occurs in approximately one of every 160,00 live births and is characterized by a a tower-shaped skull due to craniosynostosis, an underdeveloped mid-face resulting in recessed cheek bones and prominent eyes, eyes that are widely spaced and protruding, and webbed fingers and toes.

Areola: darker circle of skin surrounding the nipple of the breast.

Aesthetic plastic surgery: plastic surgery to improve the patient's looks, also called "cosmetic surgery."

Augmentation mammoplasty (or breast enlargement): breast enlargement or reconstruction by surgical insertion of a an implant.

Autologous tissue breast reconstruction: a breast reconstruction technique that uses the patient's own tissue to reconstruct a new breast.

Autologous collagen: collagen from the patients own tissue.

B

Blepharoplasty (or eye lid lift): surgery to removes excess skin, fat and muscle from the upper and lower eye lids to reshape the eye.

C

Camptodactyly: the isolated congenital flexion deformity of the proximal interphalangeal (PIP) joint.

Cannula: a hollow tube with a sharp, retractable inner core that can be inserted into a vein, artery, or other body cavity to introduce or withdraw substances.

Capsular contracture: scar tissue that forms inside the breast following breast surgery.

Carpenter's Syndrome: a very rare craniofacial birth defect that is characterized by a tower-shaped skull, webbed or additional fingers or toes, underdeveloped jaw, highly arched palate, widely spaced eyes, and/or low-set, deformed ears, reduced height, obesity, and mental deficiency. Half of patients with Carpenter's Syndrome also have heart defects.

Chemical peel: the use of chemical solutions to improve the skin's texture and appearance. Peels are used to eliminate or reduce fine lines and wrinkles around the eyes and mouth, treat acne and acne scars, correct skin pigmentation problems and remove pre-cancerous skin growths.

Chondrolaryngoplasty (or Adam's apple shaving): a surgical procedure to reduce the size and subsequent appearance of the Adam's apple.

Cleft lip: a birth defect characterized by skin and tissue separation of the upper lip.

Cleft palate: a birth defect characterized by a separation in the roof of the mouth (the palate).

Clinodactyly: the permanent lateral or medial deviation or deflection of fingers.

Collagen: a white substance composed of protein found in the connective tissues of the body including skin, bone, muscle, tendon, cartilage, and other connective tissue.

Computed tomography (CT or CAT scan): a non-surgical procedure that provides cross-section images of internal organs.

Congenital plastic surgery: plastic surgery to correct birth defects.

Cosmetic plastic surgery: see aesthetic Plastic Surgery.

Craniostenosis: see Craniosynostosis.

Craniosynostosis: a congenital birth defect that occurs when the place or joint (sutures) between plates of the skull close prematurely in early infancy resulting in an abnormal skull shape.

Crouzon's Syndrome: a birth defect occurring in approximately one of every 10,000 infants born annually in the United States and characterized by craniosynostosis, a skull that is short in the front and the back, with underdeveloped cheek bones, shallow eye sockets resulting in prominent eyes, crossed and/or wide set eyes, and a flat nose.

D

Debridment: the removal of contaminated or dead tissue from a wound to avoid infection.

Dermabrasion: a surgical procedure hat uses a high speed rotating brush to remove the top layer of skin. The procedure can remove or minimize fine wrinkles and scars on the skin, depending upon the depth of dermabrasion.

Dermaplaning: a surgical technique using an instrument called a dermatome to treat deep scars or to remove skin for grafting.

Dermatologic: pertaining to the skin.

Dermatochalasis: loose hanging skin due to connective tissue disorders. Usually genetic, but can be acquired.

Dermatome: a surgical instrument used to evenly shave off surface layers of skin.

Downs Syndrome (Trisomy 21): a birth defect caused by the presence of a third twenty-first chromosome and affecting one child in every 650 births. Downs Syndrome is characterized by low-set eras, up slanting palpebral fissures, low nasal bridge and dorsum, abnormal and excessive facial fat distribution, and a protruding, enlarged tongue.

E

Ectropion: a rare condition of the eyelid in which the lining of the eyelid turns outward at the edge and is exposed.

Endoscope: a small, flexible tube with a light and a lens on the end that is used to look inside an organ or cavity such as the esophagus, stomach, duodenum, colon, or rectum.

Endoscopy: a procedure using a lighted viewing instrument called an endoscope to look inside the body.

Erythema: redness of the skin resulting from capillary congestion.

F

Facial implant: plastic surgery to place an implant in the chin, cheek or jaw to improve facial feature proportions or to enhance facial aesthetics.

Fibril: a gelatin powder compound that is mixed with a patient's own blood and is injected to plump up the skin.

Flap surgery: surgery to relocate healthy, living tissue from one part of the body to a part that is missing tissue due to injury or disease.

Forehead lift: surgery to tighten the forehead area by removing excess fat and skin.

G

Goldenhar Syndrome: a variation of Hemifacial Microsomia. Characteristics include unilateral or bilateral underdevelopment of the mandible, unilateral or bilateral microtia, unilateral or bilateral reduction in size and flattening of the maxilla (upper jaw), narrowing of the opening of the eye, and epibulbar dermoids causing vision problems.

Gortex: a thread-like material that is implanted beneath the skin to add soft-tissue support.

Gynecomastia: enlarged male breasts; a common condition that affects an estimated 40 to 60 percent of men.

H

Hematoma: blood that has collected under the skin or in an organ.

Herpes Simplex: a viral infection caused by either herpes simplex virus type 1 or 2 which cause minor to extensive blisters. Herpes simplex type 1 is the minor variety and is responsible for blisters such as cold sores. Herpes Simplex type 2 is most commonly known as genital herpes and can cause long-term problems if left untreated. Both types are contagious via direct contact with the sores or with the fluid secreted by them.

Hyperpigmentation: the abnormal increase of skin pigmentation.

Hypertrophic scars: enlarged scars.

Hypertrophic: the increase in cell size that subsequently results in the enlargement of an organ.

Hypopigmentation: low levels of melanin production that result in lighter skin due to the lack of pigment.

I

Injectable fillers (or soft tissue augmentation): a plastic surgery technique that injects fat or collagen into an area to fill wrinkles, depressions in the skin and/or scarring.

K

Keloids: scars that overgrow and take on an irregular shape due to excessive collagen during skin repair.

L

Liposuction: a procedure to remove excess fat via a suctioning system.

M

Macrodactyly: "Macro" is a common prefix meaning "large"; "dactyl" refers to the "digits," which are fingers and toes. The condition called "macrodactyly" is an excessive largeness of one or more fingers or toes.

Mammoplasty: surgery to reduce, enlarge or reshape the breast.

Mastectomy: surgery to remove all or part of the breast.

Maxillofacial: pertaining to the face and jaws.

Metaidoioplasty: the surgical transformation of female external genitals into the male counterpart.

Milia: very small, white or yellowish bumps that are firm and occur just under the surface of the skin, usually on the face.

N

Nasolabial: pertaining to the nose and the lip.

O

Otoplasty: surgery to change the shape, reduce the size, or change the placement of ears.

P

Partial abdominoplasty (or mini tummy-tuck): surgery to flatten the abdomen when fat deposits are only found below the navel.

Periorbital rhytids: wrinkled skin around the orbit of the eye.

Pfeiffer Syndrome: a birth defect characterized by a short skull, broad, short thumbs and big toes.

Phalloplasty: the construction of male external genitalia (phallus).

Polydactyly: a birth defect caused by a genetic mutation and characterized by craniosynostosis, underdeveloped mid-face , prominent eyes, wide-set and/or crossed eyes, and broad fingers and toes.

Precancerous keratosis: small skin growths that appear wart-like and can develop into skin cancer if left untreated.

R

Reconstructive plastic surgery: plastic surgery that is performed to correct abnormalities caused by accident, infection, congenital defects, disease, and tumors.

Rhinoplasty: surgery to change the appearance of the nose by surgically sculpting the bone and cartilage.

Rhytidectomy (or facelift): surgery to smooth the appearance of the face by removing excess fat, heightening facial muscles, and stretching facial skin toward the hairline.

S

Saethre-Chotzen Syndrome: a birth defect that is closely related to Crouzon's Syndrome and is characterized by craniosynostosis, underdeveloped mid-face, a short and/or broad head, prominent, crossed and/or wide-spaced eyes, drooping eyelids, low-set hairline, and webbed fingers.

Scalp reduction: a surgical technique is used to cover the bald areas at the top and back of the head during which a segment of bald scalp is removed under local anesthesia. The hair bearing skin surrounding the cut-out area is then loosened and pulled together to close the defect.

Sclerotherapy: treatment for spider veins that involves injection of an irritating solution that inflames the lining of the vein and ultimately causes the vein to cease functioning.

Septoplasty: surgery to correct deformities of the nasal septum.

Silicone pressure therapy: a silicone dressing applied to a raised scar to help soften or thin out the scar.

Skin grafts: a section of skin used to replace damaged or missing skin. The skin may come from the patient, a cadaver or it may be grown in a lab.

Subcutaneous mastectomy: the reduction of breast volume to that of a male-appearing chest.

Symphalangia: a birth defect characterized by the end-to-end fusion of bones of the hands and feet.

Syndactyly: a birth defect characterized by webbed hands or feet.

T

Thumb hypoplasia: incomplete development of the thumb.

Tissue expander: a balloon-like device that is inserted under the skin and slowly inflated so that the covering skin expands, creating extra skin for repair of another site.

TRAM (transverse rectus abdominous muscle) flap: a popular surgical technique for breast reconstruction that involves removing an area of fat, skin and muscle from the abdomen to replace the lost breast.

Treacher-Collins Syndrome (or Mandibulofacial synostosis): a birth defect resulting from an autosomal dominant gene and characterized by facial cleft, hypoplasia of the cheeks and mandible bilaterally, colobomas (scars) of the eyelids, downward-sloping palpebral fissures, poorly developed supraorbital rims and cheeks, receding chin, and malformation of the ear.

Trigger thumb: swelling of the lubricating sheath around tendons of the thumb that can eventually cause the thumb to become "locked" in a bent position.

U

Ultrasound-Assisted Lipoplasty (UAL): liposuction that uses sound waves to break up fat prior to removal by liposuction.

V

Varicose veins: twisted, distended veins just below the skin that have become enlarged from weakened veins walls. Varicose veins appear blue and can be associated with inflammation, blood clots or ulcers.

Z

Zig-Zag Plasty: a technique of excising a scar and replacing the line with a geometric broken line.

Chapter 52

Organizational Resources

Medical Accreditation Sources

American Association for
Accreditation for Ambulatory
Surgery Facilities
1202 Allanson Road
Mundelein, IL 60060
888-545-5222
http://www.aaaasf.org

American Board of Medical
Specialties
1007 Church Street, Ste. 404
Evanston, IL 60201-5913
847-491-9091
http://www.abms.org

The American Board of Plastic
Surgery, Inc.
Seven Penn Center, Ste. 400
1635 Market Street
Philadelphia, PA 19103-2204
212-587-9322
http://www.abplsurg.org

American College of Surgeons
633 North Saint Clair Street
Chicago, IL 60611-3211
312-202-5000
E-mail: Postmaster@facs.org
http://www.facs.org

Cosmetic and Reconstructive Surgery Sources

American Academy of Pediatrics
Department of Federal Affairs
601 13ᵗʰ Street NW,
Ste. 400 North
Washington, DC 20005
http://www.aap.org

American Society for
Dermatologic Surgery
930 N. Meacham Road
Schaumburg, IL 60173-6016
Consumer Hotline: 800-441-2737
http://www.asds-net.org

American Society for Surgery of the Hand
6300 North River Road, Ste. 600
Rosemont, IL 60018-4256
847-384-8300
E-mail: info@hand-surg.org
http://www.hand-surg.org

American Society of Plastic and Reconstructive Surgical Nurses
Plastic Surgery Network
3 Via Passa
San Clemente CA 92673
E-mail: Info@plastic-surgery.net

American Society of Reconstructive Microsurgery
http://www.microsurg.org

Association of Operating Room Nurses
AORN Journal
2170 South Parker Road
Ste. 300
Denver, CO 80231-5711

Foundation for Reconstructive Plastic Surgery
http://www.frps.org

Mayo Clinic
200 First St. S.W.
Rochester, MN 55905
507-284-2511
Hearing impaired (TDD): 507-284-9786
Appointments: 507-284-2111

Mayo Clinic Scottsdale
13400 E. Shea Blvd.
Scottsdale, AZ 85259
Main: 480-301-8000
Hearing Impaired (TDD): 480-301-7683
Appointment Office: 480-301-1735

Mayo Clinic Health Oasis
http://www.mayohealth.org

Mayo Foundation for Medical Education and Research
http://www.mayo.edu

Southern California Plastic Surgery Group
8920 Wilshire Blvd., Suite 326
Beverly Hills, CA 90211
310-652-9312
2360 Long Beach Blvd.
Long Beach, CA 90806
562-595-9493
E-Mail: drhicks@face-doctor.com

The American Society for Aesthetic Plastic Surgery
E-mail: info@surgery.org
http://www.surgery.org

The Plastic Surgery Information Service
American Society of Plastic Surgeons
444 East Algonquin Road
Arlington Heights, IL 60005-4664
847-228-9900
http://www.plasticsurgery.org

Facial Cosmetic and Reconstructive Surgery

American Academy of Facial
Plastic and Reconstructive
Surgery
310 S. Henry Street
Alexandria, VA 22314
703-299-9291
800-332-FACE

American Academy of
Ophthalmology
eyeNet
http://www.aao.org

American Academy of
Otolaryngology—Head and
Neck Surgery, Inc.
One Prince Street
Alexandria, VA 22314-3357
703-836-4444
http://www.entnet.org

American Association of Oral
and Maxillofacial Surgeons
9700 West Bryn Mawr Avenue
Rosemont, IL 60018-5701
847-678-6200
E-Mail: webadmin@aaoms.org

American Society for
Dermatologic Surgery
930 N. Meacham Road
Schaumburg, IL 60173-6016
Consumer Hotline: 800-441-
2737
http://www.asds-net.org

American Society of
Ophthalmic Plastic and
Reconstructive Surgery
1133 West Morse Blvd, #201
Winter Park, FL 32789

Facial Plastic & Cosmetic
Surgical Center
6300 Regional Plaza
Abilene, TX 79606
915-695-3630; 800-592-4533
E-mail: n41gt@newlook.com
http://www.newlook.com

Mayo Foundation for Medical
Education and Research
Cosmetic Surgery On-Line
http://www.mayo.edu

National Institute of Dental &
Craniofacial Research
National Institutes of Health
Bethesda, MD 20892-2190
http://www.nidr.nih.gov

The Institute of Reconstructive
Plastic Surgery
Microtia and Aural Atresia
Division
New York University Medical
Center
550 First Avenue
New York, NY 10016
212-263-5834
http://mcrcr4.med.nyu.edu/
PlasticSurg/

The Microtia and Aural Artesia Division
Institute of Reconstructive Plastic Surgery
New York University Medical Center
http://mcrcr4.med.nyu.edu/PlasticSurg/Divs/micro.htm

The Voice Center of Eastern Virginia Medical School
Randall L. Plant, MD, MS
Medical Director
Norfolk, VA 23507
http://www.voice-center.com

World Craniofacial Foundation
7777 Forest Lane, Ste. C-612
P.O. Box 515838
Dallas, TX 75251-5838
972-566-6669; 800-533-3315
http://www.craniofacial.net

Genetic Disorder Surgery Sources

Association of Birth Defects Children, Inc.
930 Woodcock Road, Ste. 225
Orlando, FL 32803
E-mail: abdc@birthdefects.org
http://www.birthdefects.org

Genetic Alliance
4301 Connecticut Avenue, NW #404
Washington, DC 20008-2304
202-966-5557
Helpline: 800-336-GENE
E-mail: info@geneticalliance.org
http://www.geneticalliance.org

National Down Syndrome Society
666 Broadway, 8th Floor
New York, NY 10012-2317
212-460-9330
http://www.ndss.org

National Organization for Rare Disorders, Inc.
P.O. Box 8923
New Fairfield, CT 06812-8923
800-999-6673
http://ww.rarediseases.org

Office of Rare Diseases
National Institutes of Health
http://rarediseases.info.nih.gov/ord

Skin-Related Sources

American Society for Dermatologic Surgery
930 N. Meacham Road
Schaumburg, IL 60173-6016
Consumer Hotline: 800-441-2737
http://www.asds-net.org

The Burn Center
640 Jackson Street
St. Paul, MN 55101
651-221-3351 or 800-922-BURN

Skin Cancer Patients' Information Page
http://www.mpip.org

Skin Cancer Zone
http://www.skin-cancer.com

Breast Cancer and Reconstruction Sources

American Cancer Society
Breast Cancer Resource Center
800-ACS-2345
http://www.cancer.org

Association of Cancer Online
Resources
http://www.acor.org

National Alliance of Breast
Cancer Organizations
9 East 37th Street
New York, NY 10016
212-889-0606
http://www.nabco.org

The Cancer Survival Toolbox
http://www.cansearch.org/pro-
grams/toolbox

Women's Cancer Network
http://www.wcn.org

Transplantation and Replantation Resources

Martin A. Entin, MD, CM, MSc
FRCSC FACS
Royal Victoria Hospital,
Montreal, Quebec
687 Pine Avenue West
Montreal, Quebec H3A 1A1
514-843-1231

Gender Surgery Sources

GRS–Gender Reassignment
Surgery in Montreal
Clinique de chiurgie esthetique
St-Joseph
1003, boul. St-Joseph Est
Monreal (Quebec) H2J 1L2
www.grsmontreal.com

The Harry Benjamin
International Gender Dysphoria
Association, Inc.
1300 South Second Street, Suite
180
Minneapolis, MN 55454
612-625-1500

Plastic Surgery News Resources

Cancer News on the Net
http://www.cancernews.com

CNN.com Health
http://www.cnn.com/HEALTH

Health Finder
http://www.healthfinder.gov

MD Linx
http://www.mdlinx.com

Medicine Net
http://www.medicinenet.com

Medscape Inc.
http://www.medscape .com

Med Serve Medical News
http://www.medserve.dk

MED WEB (Emory University)
http://www.medweb.emory.edu

National Library of Medicine
National Institutes of Health
http://www.nlm.nih.gov

P/S/L Consulting Group, Inc.
1250 René-Lévesque Ouest,
Suite 3200
Montréal, Québec, H3B 4W8
http://www.pslgroup.com

Reuters Health Information
http://www.reutershealth.com

No-Cost Reconstructive Surgery Sources

Healing the Children
http:www.northeast.net/HTC

Pub Med Central
National Institutes of Health
http://
www.pubmedcentral.nih.gov

Operation Smile
6435 Tidewater Drive
Norfolk, VA 23509
757-321-SMILE (7645)
http://operationsmile.org

Plasticos Foundation
7677 Center Avenue, Ste. 40
Huntington Beach, CA 92647
714-902-1111
E-mail:
plasticosfoundation@yahoo.com
http://
wwwplasticosfoundation.org

Rotaplast International
415-538-8120
http://www.rotaplast.org

Small World Foundation
7710 N.W. 71st Court, Ste. 206
Fort Lauderdale, FL 33321
800-965-4793
E-mail: info@smallworld.org
http://www.smallworld.org

The Foundation for
Reconstructive Plastic Surgery
212-794-1234
http://www.frps.org

Uplift Internationale
http://
wwwupliftinternationale.org

WebMedLit
http://
webmedlit.silverplatter.com

Insurance Information Sources

INSURE.COM
76 LaSalle Road
West Hartford, CT 06107
860-233-2800
http://www.insure.com

Medline Plus
National Library of Medicine
National Institutes of Health
http://
www.medlineplus.nlm.nih.gov

The Plastic Surgery Education
Foundation
American Society of Plastic
Surgeons
444 East Algonquin Road
Arlington Heights, IL 60005-4664
847-228-9900
http://www.plasticsurgery.org

Additional Information Sources

Argus Clearinghouse
http://www.clearinghouse.net

California Society of Plastic
Surgeons Alliance
525 Spruce Street
San Francisco, CA 94118
415-668-9496
http://www.ca-soc-
plasticsurgeons.com/
csps_alliance1.cgi

Health On the Net Foundation
http://www.hon.ch

Health Web
http://healthweb.org

Pub Med Central
National Institutes of Health
http://
www.pubmedcentral.nih.gov

Science.komm
http://www.sciencekomm.at

Chapter 53

Insurance Information

Contents

Section 53.1

Insurance Coverage: A Patient's Guide

American Society of Plastic Surgeons, reprinted from the
Plastic Surgery Information Service at http://www.plasticsurgery.org.
© 1993; reprinted with permission.

Staying Informed about Your Health Care Costs

As you plan for plastic surgery, you will probably learn a lot about
what will happen in the operating room and discuss with your plastic surgeon how you will look and feel afterward. However, another
important part of being an informed patient is knowing about the costs
associated with surgery, and how these costs will be paid.

The American Society of Plastic Surgeons (ASPS) has prepared this
information to assist you in better understanding health insurance
benefits for plastic surgery. It is intended to answer basic questions
and guide you in communicating effectively with your plastic surgeon's
office staff and your insurance carrier. It won't answer all of your
questions, because a lot depends on individual circumstances and your
own insurance. Be sure to contact your insurance company or your
employer's Human Resources/Benefits department with any questions
you have about coverage for specific services.

About Plastic Surgery

Derived from the Greek word "plastikos," meaning to mold or give
form, the specialty of plastic surgery encompasses two general categories:

- Reconstructive surgery is performed on abnormal structures of the
  body, caused by congenital defects, developmental abnormalities,
  trauma, infection, tumors, or disease. It is generally performed to
  improve function, but may also be done to approximate a normal
  appearance.

- Cosmetic surgery is performed to reshape normal structures of the
  body in order to improve the patient's appearance and self-esteem.

326

• Definitions as adopted by the American Medical Association and the American Society of Plastic Surgeons (ASPS).

What's Covered

Your insurance policy is an agreement between you and your insurance company. In contrast, an agreement on services and fees is an agreement between you and your plastic surgeon. When you have surgery, you become responsible for payment of the doctor's fees. Coverage for services and levels of payment by your insurance company depend on the terms of the contract between you and your insurance company. You are responsible for any amounts not covered by your plan.

Reconstructive surgery is generally covered by most health insurance policies, although coverage for specific procedures and levels of coverage may vary greatly.

Cosmetic surgery, however, is usually not covered by health insurance because it is elective. Cosmetic surgery is your choice and not considered a medical necessity.

There are a number of "gray areas" in coverage for plastic surgery that sometimes require special consideration by an insurance carrier. These areas usually involve surgical operations which may be reconstructive or cosmetic, depending on each patient's situation. For example, eyelid surgery (blepharoplasty)—a procedure normally performed to achieve cosmetic improvement—may be covered if the eyelids are drooping severely and obscuring a patient's vision. Or, nose surgery (rhinoplasty and/or septoplasty) may be covered if it will correct a defect that causes breathing difficulties.

In assessing whether the procedure will be covered by the patient's insurance contract, the carrier looks at the primary reason the procedure is being performed: is it for relief of symptoms or for cosmetic improvement? If a procedure is within these "gray areas," insurance companies often require prior authorization or approval before the surgery is performed and/or extra documentation after surgery to determine how much of the cost of your care they will cover.

Reading Your Own Policy

It's important to understand what's included in your policy before you advance too far in planning surgery. Some policies provide coverage for many plastic surgery procedures while others are more limited in coverage. Read your policy and benefits manual carefully and

327

discuss any questions you may have with your insurance plan manager.

There are three typical cost sharing options:

- a deductible, is the total amount of covered medical expenses that must be paid by the patient before the insurance company begins paying benefits. Examples of standard deductibles are $100, $250, or $500. After this requirement is reached, the insurer will begin paying according to terms of the contract—often 75 percent to 85 percent of covered medical costs. The patient is responsible for any remaining balance.

- a flat-rate co-payment, reflects a defined share of covered medical costs that the patient pays, with the insurance carrier paying an amount based on the patient's policy. For example, when the patient pays $15 of any office visit charge or $3 for any prescription, the insurance carrier is responsible for the balance.

- a percentage-based co-payment, reflects a percentage share of covered medical costs that the patient pays, with the insurance company paying an amount based on the patient's policy. Examples are: 20 percent of the office visit charge—$10 of a $50 charge, $12 of a $60 charge, etc. Typically, this co-payment arrangement includes a deductible and may have other variations.

Your benefits administrator will be able to explain these points to you. Be certain that all patient financial responsibilities are understood before having surgery. If you can calculate your costs based on the terms of your insurance plan, there will be no misunderstanding later of your obligation.

Example One

A woman is planning to undergo hand surgery, the surgical fee will be $2,000. Her plan has a $250 annual deductible, and will cover 80 percent of her covered medical costs. Because she has paid only $70 so far this year in covered medical expenses, she must pay the first $180 of the covered costs of the hand surgery to satisfy her plan's $250 deductible. If her plan cost's share is a percentage-based co-payment of 80 percent to 20 percent, the carrier will pay 80 percent of the covered costs of the procedure. Once that is settled, she must pay for 20 percent of the covered costs, plus any costs for which the insurance plan denies coverage.

If the patient's insurance plan covered the full surgical fee, the cost sharing would look like this:

Reconstructive Hand Surgery: $2,000
Balance of deductible: $180 ($250 - $70)

$1,820
Insurance coverage: $1,820 x 80% = $1,456
Patient payment: $2,000 - $1,456 = $544

The $544 is the patient's responsibility under the percentage-based co-payment arrangement.

Example Two

A different scenario occurs if the patient has met the deductible and the plan covers the full surgical fee. Then the math might look like this:

Reconstructive Hand Surgery: $2,000
Percentage-based agreement: $1,600 (80%)
Patient payment: $400

The patient's responsibility is, in this example, $400.

Example Three

If the patient's insurance has a flat-rate co-payment plan for covered medical services with no other limiting conditions and the co-payment rate is $15, then the surgical cost might be paid as follows:

Reconstructive Hand Surgery: $2,000
Contracted patient co-payment: $15
Balance paid by insurance: $1,985

Example Four

With a coordination of benefits or dual coverage, the hand surgery patient is also covered under her spouse's insurance, and the benefits of both plans may be coordinated to cover more of the cost of the surgery. With dual coverage, the patient's carrier is considered the primary insurer. Coverage under a percentage-based co-payment is 80 percent of the cost of surgery. The secondary insurer, her spouse's plan, may cover the remaining 20 percent, depending on the specific terms of the spouse's policy.

After the primary insurer has paid its share, it will send the patient an "explanation of benefits" statement, including the date of service, the doctor's charges and/or hospital covered charges, the amounts and payment dispersal dates. If the patient is covered under only one plan, she must pay the unpaid balance. With dual coverage, the secondary insurer may pay some or all of the remaining balance. Usually, the secondary insurer will not pay for any portion of the remaining balance until a copy of the primary insurer's benefits statement is received.

The above illustrate examples of coverage. The amount billed to your insurance by your physician may not be the actual amount on which reimbursement is calculated; your insurance plan may assign a lesser fee for the procedure. Where a physician has agreed to be a contracted provider, these illustrations will not necessarily apply.

Your particular situation will:

- reflect the coverage and cost-sharing agreement of your insurance plan;

- the deductible and any amount of the deductible that you have already met;

- and any dual coverage available if you are also carried on your spouse's or another secondary plan.

Understanding your policy and your responsibility for payment is essential. Securing approval of medical services and fees by your insurance carrier prior to surgery will prevent any misunderstanding of coverage and responsibility for payment after your care is complete.

Beginning the Process

When you visit your plastic surgeon's office for the first time, bring your insurance card with you. If you are eligible for coverage under another plan, bring this insurance card with you as well. With verification of this information on file, the plastic surgeon's office staff may bill your health care plan directly for covered services.

Once you and your plastic surgeon have agreed on the specifics of your care and the fees, it's likely that your plastic surgeon will assist in determining if your care is indeed covered by your insurance plan.

Your plastic surgeon will probably send a pre-authorization letter to your insurance carrier, explaining the procedure, listing the ICD-9 (diagnosis) and CPT (procedure) codes, the surgical fee, place of service, and anesthesia. The pre-authorization letter will request authorization to proceed with your surgery and an indication of the level of coverage provided by your policy. Before giving the "go-ahead" to proceed with surgery, the insurance company will review your case to ensure that the procedure is medically necessary based on the insurance carrier's guidelines of medical necessity.

During this review period, make sure you have a clear understanding of the costs and fees, and determine the portion you'll be expected to pay. Remember, if a hospital stay is also required, a number of other costs will be involved.

Keep accurate notes of all communication with the insurance company and your plastic surgeon, and make a personal file to keep copies of completed insurance forms and every letter sent or received. Keep your file in a safe place in case papers are lost in the insurance process or the mail or you need to reference anything about your surgery.

The Appeals Process: Another Chance at Coverage

If your insurance company does not authorize payment for your reconstructive surgery, or if it agrees to pay only a small percentage of a claim, you may choose to appeal the decision.

Before beginning this process, carefully read your policy or benefits booklet. Make sure there is nothing in the plan that specifically excludes the type of care you received or are scheduled to receive.

In appealing the decision, your first step is to write a letter to the insurance company representative (usually the claims supervisor) who signed the notification of denial. In the letter, explain why you feel the procedure should be covered and ask that your request be reviewed by a plastic surgeon certified by the American Board of Plastic Surgery.

Your appeal letter should also request a full explanation of why coverage is being denied or paid at a reduced level. Request that the claims supervisor send you a copy of the specific statement—drawn from the policy or from the benefits booklet—that explains why your coverage is limited or denied. Attach a copy of the denial notification and a copy of your doctor's pre-authorization letter to again provide the statement of your surgeon's fee, the applicable billing codes, and an ASPS Position Paper specific to your procedure. Position papers are available from your plastic surgeon.

If you receive a vague response, or an explanation that "your policy does not cover this type of surgery," you have the right to see that policy language in writing. Make certain that these policy restrictions were in place when you first began your contract with the health plan and started paying premiums. If the restrictions were not initially in place, you may have the right to coverage under the insurance laws of your state.

Many patients find it helpful to send a duplicate mailing of their appeal letter to the insurance commissioner of their home state for indemnity insurance, or to the department of corporations if you are covered under a managed care plan such as a health maintenance organization (HMO). This should include a brief cover letter explaining the trouble you are having and asking for assistance.

If your insurance company responds favorably to your appeal, notify the commissioner of your successful appeal efforts with a second letter.

Paying for Cosmetic Surgery

Your plastic surgeon practices in an ethical manner and will submit claims to insurance carriers only for valid reconstructive plastic surgery. Any attempt to misrepresent a cosmetic procedure as reconstructive is unethical. Cosmetic procedures are elective, and payment is the responsibility of the patient.

Some plastic surgeons accept major credit cards or offer financing programs that allow patients to make manageable monthly payments for cosmetic surgery. Ask your surgeon's office staff if any such programs are available.

Glossary of Terms

ASPS Position Paper: a written statement by the American Society of Plastic Surgeons detailing the background and medical indications for reconstructive and cosmetic surgical procedures. Position papers covering the most common plastic surgery procedures are available.

Co-payment: in a contract with a health plan, the portion of covered medical costs that the patient pays. In a typical plan, the patient's co-payment may be based on a percentage or a flat rate.

Coordination of Benefits: occurs when a patient is eligible for coverage by more than one insurance plan. The benefits of the plans are coordinated so that the patient may receive up to 100-percent coverage for his or her medical costs.

CPT Code: a code number used to identify medical services. Developed by the American Medical Association, "CPT" stands for Current Procedural Terminology. CPT codes are used by physicians in billing for services performed.

Deductible: the total amount of covered medical-care expenses that must be paid by the patient, usually on an annual basis, before the insurance company begins paying benefits.

Exclusion: a condition or circumstance for which a health plan does not provide benefits.

ICD-9 Code: a code that indicates the diagnosis-illness, disease or trauma-for which care was rendered. "ICD" stands for International Classification of Disease. Diagnosis codes must correlate correctly with CPT codes for an insurance carrier to consider payment.

Pre-authorization letter: a letter written by a physician to an insurance company prior to surgery. It explains in detail the procedure a patient plans to have and requests confirmation that the patient is covered, the planned services are covered, and the level of coverage for the planned services.

Pre-determination: a review process conducted by an insurance company to verify the medical necessity of a planned procedure or treatment. Pre-determination is often a condition of plan payment.

The American Society of Plastic Surgeons (ASPS) represents approximately 5,000 plastic surgeons in the United States and Canada and is the largest organization of plastic surgeons in the world. Requirements for membership include certification by the American Board of Plastic Surgery (ABPS).

As the umbrella organization for the specialty, ASPS represents 97 percent of the board-certified plastic surgeons practicing in the United States and Canada. It serves as the primary educational resource for plastic surgeons and as their voice on socioeconomic issues. ASPS is recognized by the American Medical Association (AMA), the American College of Surgeons (ACS) and other organizations of specialty societies.

American Society of Plastic Surgeons, 444 East Algonquin Road, Arlington Heights, Illinois 60005-4664, 847-228-9900.

Section 53.2

State Laws—Breast Reconstruction: Insurance Coverage Required for Post-Mastectomy Reconstruction if Mastectomy is Covered

American Society of Plastic Surgeons, reprinted from
The Plastic Surgery Information Service at www.plasticsurgery.org.
© 1998; reprinted with permission.

The following information was completed in 1998 and is the most recent available. However, more recent legislation may have been enacted at the state level which could alter insurance coverage for breast reconstruction surgery. For the most current information on your state's laws, contact the Plastic Surgery Information Service at (800) 635-0635.

Arizona—covers surgical services for breast reconstruction, and at least two external post-operative prostheses.

Arkansas—enacted in 1997; covers prosthetic devices and reconstructive surgery.

California—enacted in 1978, covers prosthetic devices or reconstructive surgery incident to mastectomy, including restoring symmetry; law was amended in 1991 to include coverage for pre-1980 mastectomies.

Connecticut—enacted in 1987; covers at least a yearly benefit of $500 for reconstructive surgery, $300 for prosthesis, and $300 for surgical removal of each breast due to tumor.

Florida—covers initial prosthetic device and reconstructive surgery incident to mastectomy; 1997 amendment states that the surgery must be in a manner chosen by the treating physician, and specifies that surgery to reestablish symmetry between the two breasts is covered.

Illinois—enacted in 1981; covers initial prosthetic device and reconstructive surgery incident to post-1981 mastectomies.

Indiana—enacted in 1997; covers prosthetic devices and reconstructive surgery following a mastectomy.

Kentucky—enacted in 1998; covers all stages of breast reconstruction surgery following a mastectomy that resulted from breast cancer.

Louisiana—enacted in 1997; covers reconstructive surgery following a mastectomy, including reconstruction of the other breast to produce a symmetrical appearance.

Maine—enacted in 1995; covers both breast on which surgery was performed and the other breast if patient elects reconstruction, in the manner chosen by the patient and physician.

Maryland—enacted in 1996; requires coverage for reconstructive surgery resulting from a mastectomy, including surgery performed on a non-diseased breast to establish symmetry.

Michigan—enacted in 1989; covers breast cancer rehabilitative services, delivered on an inpatient or outpatient basis, including reconstructive plastic surgery and physical therapy.

Minnesota—enacted in 1980; covers all reconstructive surgery incidental to or following injury, sickness or other diseases of the involved part, or congenital defect for a child.

Missouri—enacted in 1997; covers prosthetic devices and reconstructive surgery necessary to achieve symmetry.

Montana—enacted in 1997; eff. Jan. 1, 1998; covers reconstructive surgery following a mastectomy resulting from breast cancer, including all stages of one reconstructive surgery on the non-diseased breast to establish symmetry, and costs of any prostheses.

Nevada—enacted in 1983; covers at least two prosthetic devices and reconstructive surgery incident to mastectomy. The law was amended in 1989 to cover surgery to reestablish symmetry.

New Hampshire—enacted in 1997; eff. Jan. 1, 1998; covers breast reconstruction, including surgery and reconstruction of the other breast to produce a symmetrical appearance, in the manner chosen by the patient and physician.

New Jersey—enacted in 1985; covers reconstructive breast surgery, including cost of prostheses. The law was amended in 1997 to extend coverage to reconstructive surgery to achieve and restore symmetry.

New York—enacted in 1997, eff. Jan. 1, 1998; covers breast reconstruction following mastectomy, including reconstruction on a healthy breast required to achieve reasonable symmetry, in the manner determined to be appropriate by the attending physician and the patient.

N. Carolina—enacted in 1997; covers reconstructive breast surgery, including reconstructive surgery performed on a non-diseased breast to establish symmetry.

Oklahoma—enacted in 1997; eff. Jan. 1, 1998; covers reconstructive breast surgery performed as a result of a partial or total mastectomy, including all stages of reconstructive surgery performed on a non-diseased breast to establish symmetry.

Pennsylvania—enacted in 1997; covers prosthetic devices and breast reconstruction, including surgery of the opposite breast to achieve symmetry, within six years of the mastectomy date.

Rhode Island—enacted in 1996; covers prosthetic devices and reconstructive surgery to restore and achieve symmetry incident to a mastectomy. Surgery must be performed within 18 months of the original mastectomy.

South Carolina—enacted in 1998; eff. Jan. 1, 1999; covers prosthetic devices and breast reconstruction, including the non-diseased breast, if determined medically necessary by the patient's attending physician with the approval of the insurer.

Tennessee—enacted in 1997; eff. July 1, 1997; covers both breast on which surgery was performed and the other breast if patient elects reconstruction, in the manner chosen by the patient and physician.

Texas—enacted in 1997; eff. Sept. 1, 1997; covers breast reconstruction, including procedures to restore and achieve symmetry, for contracts delivered, issued for delivery or renewed on or after Jan. 1, 1998.

Virginia—enacted in 1998; eff. July 1, 1998; covers reconstructive breast surgery performed coincident with a mastectomy performed for breast cancer or following the mastectomy, and surgery performed to reestablish symmetry between the two breasts.

Washington—enacted in 1983; covers reconstructive breast surgery if mastectomy resulted from disease, illness or injury. The law was amended in 1996 to include surgery to reestablish symmetry.

Wisconsin—enacted in 1997; covers breast reconstruction of the affected tissue incident to mastectomy and specifies that such surgery is not to be considered cosmetic.

Section 53.3

Congress Requires Breast Reconstruction

Among the many provisions included in the 40-pound Omnibus Budget Bill that passed Congress is one that requires health insurance companies to cover the cost of reconstructive breast surgery for women who have undergone mastectomies. Introduced by Sen. Alfonse D'Amato (R-N.Y.) and supported by a number of lawmakers, including Sen. Diane Feinstein (D-Calif.) and Sen. Edward Kennedy (D-Mass.), the provision passed both the House and Senate, and was signed by President Clinton on Oct. 21 (1998).

So far, 29 states have passed laws requiring insurance companies to pay for breast-reconstruction surgery. However, not all health plans are subject to state regulation. The federal provision will fill in those regulatory gaps by amending ERISA, the law that governs all health insurance and employee health benefit programs.

Advocates for the health insurance industry characterize the provision as well-intended but misguided. Chip Kahn, president of the Health Insurance Association of America, called the measure "yet another example of Congressional 'body part' language compelling health plans to devote scarce resources to one course of treatment, potentially at the expense of other worthy services."

Not surprisingly, the American Society of Plastic and Reconstructive Surgeons applauded the provision. A recent survey by the professional group found that 84 percent of member physicians had patients who were denied coverage for breast-reconstruction surgery following a mastectomy.

Section 53.4

Survey Reveals Poor Coverage for Kids' Plastic Surgery

"Poor Coverage for Kids' Plastic Surgery: American Society of Plastic and Reconstructive Surgeons Survey Reveals Insurance Denial or Trouble in Getting Coverage for Deformities and other Facial Defects," in *USA Today (Magazine)*, February 1998 vol. 126, no.2633, p. 8(2). © 1998 Society for the Advancement of Education; reprinted with permission.

In a survey conducted by the American Society of Plastic and Reconstructive Surgeons (ASPRS), more than half of its members who were polled reported insurance denial or trouble obtaining coverage of procedures for deformities, disfigurements, and congenital defects in children. According to the ASPRS survey, the most often denied procedures are associated with nose reshaping for congenital nasal deformities related to cleft lip and craniofacial deformity, repair of an abnormally small outer ear, and cleft lip repair.

"Insurance coverage denial for pediatric plastic surgery procedures is a symptom of the broader issues plaguing the state of medical care in this country today. From decreased hospital stays to increased insurance denials for procedures traditionally covered, insurance companies, rather than medical professionals, are determining the quality of patient care," says ASPRS president Dennis Lynch.

The American Medical Association (AMA) has passed a resolution stating that treatment of a minor child's congenital or developmental deformity or disorder due to trauma or malignant disease should be covered by all insurers. Moreover, such coverage should include treatment that, in the opinion of the treating physician, is medically necessary to return the patient to a more normal appearance (even if the procedure does not affect materially the function of that body part), and such insurability should be portable—i.e., not denied as a pre-existing condition if the patients insurance coverage changes before treatment has been initiated or completed.

AMA Board of Trustees member Edward Hill of Tupelo, Miss., notes that plastic surgery that allows a child to have a normal appearance—even if it doesn't improve bodily function—is important for social acceptance. "What about mental function? What about psychological function? Can you imagine the life of a child with a gross deformity, which can be repaired, as far as the mental health concerns for the rest of their lives? We have some real concerns with that."

Index

Index

Page numbers followed by 'n' indicate a footnote. Page numbers in *italics* indicate a table or illustration.

A

AAAAPSF *see* American Association for Accreditation of Ambulatory Plastic Surgery Facilities

AAFPRS *see* American Academy of Facial Plastic and Reconstructive Surgery

abdominal surgery, insurance coverage 9

abdominoplasty ("tummy tuck") 159–62
  average costs *19*
  complications 160
  defined 309
  endoscopy 66–67
  partial, defined 314
  statistics *13*, *17*

ABPS *see* American Board of Plastic Surgery

acne scars 79, 107
  chemical peels 112
  dermabrasion 115
  see also scars

ACS *see* American Cancer Society

Adam's apple shaving *see* chondrolaryngoplasty

adolescents
  breast reduction 145
  plastic surgery 28, 31–34

Advanced Tissue Sciences, Inc. 229, 231

aesthetic facial surgery 59

aesthetic plastic surgery
  adolescents 31–34
  defined 309

"Aesthetic Plastic Surgery for Teen-agers: When is it Appropriate?" 31n

age factor
  cosmetic surgery *12–13*
  plastic surgery 6

Alberisio, A. 276

alexandrite lasers *see* lasers

allografts 217, 219, 227

AMA *see* American Medical Association

ambulatory phlebectomy 165

American Academy of Facial and Reconstructive Plastic Surgeons 35n

American Academy of Facial Plastic and Reconstructive Surgery (AAFPRS)
  autologous fibroblast grafting 79
  blepharoplasty 121n
  contact information 319
  motivations for surgery 36
  rhinoplasty 129n

343

"Breast Cancer Network Update -
Breast Reconstruction" 253n
breast development, abnormal 8
breast enlargement *see* mammoplasty: augmentation
breastfeeding
breast implants 47, 136
breast reduction 145
breast lift *see* mastoplexy
breast reconstruction *see* mammoplasty: reconstruction
"Breast reconstruction" (Schain) 277
breast reduction *see* mammoplasty:
reduction
Breidenbach, Warren 279, 280, 281
Breu, Giovanna 281
Bronaugh, Robert L. 231
browlifts *see* forehead lifts
Brown, James Barrett 219
Bryan, Lauran 239
Buncke, Harry 284, 285, 290
"Burn Care and Rehabilitation Principles and Practice" (Richard, et al.)
224
The Burn Center, contact information
320
burns
artificial skin 225–32
grafts 21, 74
statistics *14*
Bushnell, S. S. 276
buttock lifts
average costs *18*
statistics *12, 16*

C

cadaver skin 217, 219–20, 227
see also artificial skin; pig skin;
skin grafts
cafe-au-lait spots 57
Cahn, Frederick 229
Cajal, Ramon Y. 290
calcium deposits, breast implants 47,
136
calf implants, statistics *16*
California Society of Plastic Surgeons
Alliance, contact information 323

camptodactyly *202*, 206, *207*
defined 310
Canadian Journal of Plastic Surgery
283n
Cancer 276, 277
Cancer News on the Net, website 321
Cancer Survival Toolbox, website
321
cannula 157
defined 310
Canthopexy Pre-op *41*
canthoplasty *40*
Capelli, M. 276
Caplan, Arthur 280
capsular contracture 136
breast implants 46–47
capsular contracture, defined 310
carbolic acid 112
carbon dioxide (CO_2) lasers *see* lasers
Card, I. C. 276
carpal tunnel release, endoscopy 68
Carpenter's syndrome 193–94
defined 310
CAT scan *see* computerized axial tomography
Cederna, P. S. 276
certification, plastic surgeons 4, 23,
317
Chaglassian, T. 277
Chang, P. 276
cheek implants 125
adolescents 33
average costs *18*
statistics *12, 16*
chemical peels 109, 111–14, 116
average costs *18*
complications 113
defined 310
statistics *12, 16*
Ch'en, Chung Wei 285, 286, 289, 291
children
clefts 169–72
ear shaping surgery 133
insurance coverage 338–39
plastic surgery 28, 237–40
chin augmentation 125, 130
adolescents 34
average costs *18*
statistics *12, 16*

Health Reference Series
COMPLETE CATALOG

AIDS Sourcebook, 1st Edition

Basic Information about AIDS and HIV Infection, Featuring Historical and Statistical Data, Current Research, Prevention, and Other Special Topics of Interest for Persons Living with AIDS

Along with Source Listings for Further Assistance

Edited by Karen Bellenir and Peter D. Dresser. 831 pages. 1995. 0-7808-0031-1. $78.

"One strength of this book is its practical emphasis. The intended audience is the lay reader . . . useful as an educational tool for health care providers who work with AIDS patients. Recommended for public libraries as well as hospital or academic libraries that collect consumer materials."
—*Bulletin of the Medical Library Association, Jan '96*

"This is the most comprehensive volume of its kind on an important medical topic. Highly recommended for all libraries."　—*Reference Book Review, '96*

"Very useful reference for all libraries."
—*Choice, Association of College and Research Libraries, Oct '95*

"There is a wealth of information here that can provide much educational assistance. It is a must book for all libraries and should be on the desk of each and every congressional leader. Highly recommended."
—*AIDS Book Review Journal, Aug '95*

"Recommended for most collections."
—*Library Journal, Jul '95*

AIDS Sourcebook, 2nd Edition

Basic Consumer Health Information about Acquired Immune Deficiency Syndrome (AIDS) and Human Immunodeficiency Virus (HIV) Infection, Featuring Updated Statistical Data, Reports on Recent Research and Prevention Initiatives, and Other Special Topics of Interest for Persons Living with AIDS, Including New Antiretroviral Treatment Options, Strategies for Combating Opportunistic Infections, Information about Clinical Trials, and More

Along with a Glossary of Important Terms and Resource Listings for Further Help and Information

Edited by Karen Bellenir. 751 pages. 1999. 0-7808-0225-X. $78.

"Highly recommended."
—*American Reference Books Annual, 2000*

"Excellent sourcebook. This continues to be a highly recommended book. There is no other book that provides as much information as this book provides."
—*AIDS Book Review Journal, Dec-Jan 2000*

"Recommended reference source."
—*Booklist, American Library Association, Dec '99*

"A solid text for college-level health libraries."
—*The Bookwatch, Aug '99*

Cited in *Reference Sources for Small and Medium-Sized Libraries, American Library Association, 1999*

Alcoholism Sourcebook

Basic Consumer Health Information about the Physical and Mental Consequences of Alcohol Abuse, Including Liver Disease, Pancreatitis, Wernicke-Korsakoff Syndrome (Alcoholic Dementia), Fetal Alcohol Syndrome, Heart Disease, Kidney Disorders, Gastrointestinal Problems, and Immune System Compromise and Featuring Facts about Addiction, Detoxification, Alcohol Withdrawal, Recovery, and the Maintenance of Sobriety

Along with a Glossary and Directories of Resources for Further Help and Information

Edited by Karen Bellenir. 613 pages. 2000. 0-7808-0325-6. $78.

"Recommended reference source."
—*Booklist, American Library Association, Dec '00*

"Presents a wealth of information on alcohol use and abuse and its effects on the body and mind, treatment, and prevention." —*SciTech Book News, Dec '00*

"Important new health guide which packs in the latest consumer information about the problems of alcoholism." —*Reviewer's Bookwatch, Nov '00*

SEE ALSO Drug Abuse Sourcebook, Substance Abuse Sourcebook

Allergies Sourcebook

Basic Information about Major Forms and Mechanisms of Common Allergic Reactions, Sensitivities, and Intolerances, Including Anaphylaxis, Asthma, Hives and Other Dermatologic Symptoms, Rhinitis, and Sinusitis

Along with Their Usual Triggers Like Animal Fur, Chemicals, Drugs, Dust, Foods, Insects, Latex, Pollen, and Poison Ivy, Oak, and Sumac; Plus Information on Prevention, Identification, and Treatment

Edited by Allan R. Cook. 611 pages. 1997. 0-7808-0036-2. $78.

Alternative Medicine Sourcebook

Basic Consumer Health Information about Alternatives to Conventional Medicine, Including Acupressure, Acupuncture, Aromatherapy, Ayurveda, Bioelectromagnetics, Environmental Medicine, Essence

Therapy, Food and Nutrition Therapy, Herbal Therapy, Homeopathy, Imaging, Massage, Naturopathy, Reflexology, Relaxation and Meditation, Sound Therapy, Vitamin and Mineral Therapy, and Yoga, and More

Edited by Allan R. Cook. 737 pages. 1999. 0-7808-0200-4. $78.

"Recommended reference source."
    —*Booklist, American Library Association, Feb '00*

"A great addition to the reference collection of every type of library." —*American Reference Books Annual, 2000*

∎

Alzheimer's, Stroke & 29 Other Neurological Disorders Sourcebook, 1st Edition

Basic Information for the Layperson on 31 Diseases or Disorders Affecting the Brain and Nervous System, First Describing the Illness, Then Listing Symptoms, Diagnostic Methods, and Treatment Options, and Including Statistics on Incidences and Causes

Edited by Frank E. Bair. 579 pages. 1993. 1-55888-748-2. $78.

"Nontechnical reference book that provides reader-friendly information."
    —*Family Caregiver Alliance Update, Winter '96*

"Should be included in any library's patient education section." —*American Reference Books Annual, 1994*

"Written in an approachable and accessible style. Recommended for patient education and consumer health collections in health science center and public libraries." —*Academic Library Book Review, Dec '93*

"It is very handy to have information on more than thirty neurological disorders under one cover, and there is no recent source like it." —*Reference Quarterly, American Library Association, Fall '93*

SEE ALSO Brain Disorders Sourcebook

∎

Alzheimer's Disease Sourcebook, 2nd Edition

Basic Consumer Health Information about Alzheimer's Disease, Related Disorders, and Other Dementias, Including Multi-Infarct Dementia, AIDS-Related Dementia, Alcoholic Dementia, Huntington's Disease, Delirium, and Confusional States

Along with Reports Detailing Current Research Efforts in Prevention and Treatment, Long-Term Care Issues, and Listings of Sources for Additional Help and Information

Edited by Karen Bellenir. 524 pages. 1999. 0-7808-0223-3. $78.

"Provides a wealth of useful information not otherwise available in one place. This resource is recommended for all types of libraries."
    —*American Reference Books Annual, 2000*

"Recommended reference source."
    —*Booklist, American Library Association, Oct '99*

Arthritis Sourcebook

Basic Consumer Health Information about Specific Forms of Arthritis and Related Disorders, Including Rheumatoid Arthritis, Osteoarthritis, Gout, Polymyalgia Rheumatica, Psoriatic Arthritis, Spondyloarthropathies, Juvenile Rheumatoid Arthritis, and Juvenile Ankylosing Spondylitis

Along with Information about Medical, Surgical, and Alternative Treatment Options, and Including Strategies for Coping with Pain, Fatigue, and Stress

Edited by Allan R. Cook. 550 pages. 1998. 0-7808-0201-2. $78.

". . . accessible to the layperson."
    —*Reference and Research Book News, Feb '99*

∎

Asthma Sourcebook

Basic Consumer Health Information about Asthma, Including Symptoms, Traditional and Nontraditional Remedies, Treatment Advances, Quality-of-Life Aids, Medical Research Updates, and the Role of Allergies, Exercise, Age, the Environment, and Genetics in the Development of Asthma

Along with Statistical Data, a Glossary, and Directories of Support Groups, and Other Resources for Further Information

Edited by Annemarie S. Muth. 628 pages. 2000. 0-7808-0381-7. $78.

"Highly recommended." —*The Bookwatch, Jan '01*

∎

Back & Neck Disorders Sourcebook

Basic Information about Disorders and Injuries of the Spinal Cord and Vertebrae, Including Facts on Chiropractic Treatment, Surgical Interventions, Paralysis, and Rehabilitation

Along with Advice for Preventing Back Trouble

Edited by Karen Bellenir. 548 pages. 1997. 0-7808-0202-0. $78.

"The strength of this work is its basic, easy-to-read format. Recommended."
    —*Reference and User Services Quarterly, American Library Association, Winter '97*

∎

Blood & Circulatory Disorders Sourcebook

Basic Information about Blood and Its Components, Anemias, Leukemias, Bleeding Disorders, and Circulatory Disorders, Including Aplastic Anemia, Thalassemia, Sickle-Cell Disease, Hemochromatosis, Hemophilia, Von Willebrand Disease, and Vascular Diseases

Along with a Special Section on Blood Transfusions and Blood Supply Safety, a Glossary, and Source Listings for Further Help and Information

Edited by Karen Bellenir and Linda M. Shin. 554 pages. 1998. 0-7808-0203-9. $78.

"Recommended reference source."
—*Booklist, American Library Association, Feb '99*

"An important reference sourcebook written in simple language for everyday, non-technical users. "
—*Reviewer's Bookwatch, Jan '99*

■

Brain Disorders Sourcebook

Basic Consumer Health Information about Strokes, Epilepsy, Amyotrophic Lateral Sclerosis (ALS/Lou Gehrig's Disease), Parkinson's Disease, Brain Tumors, Cerebral Palsy, Headache, Tourette Syndrome, and More

Along with Statistical Data, Treatment and Rehabilitation Options, Coping Strategies, Reports on Current Research Initiatives, a Glossary, and Resource Listings for Additional Help and Information

Edited by Karen Bellenir. 481 pages. 1999. 0-7808-0229-2. $78.

"Belongs on the shelves of any library with a consumer health collection." —*E-Streams, Mar '00*

"Recommended reference source."
—*Booklist, American Library Association, Oct '99*

SEE ALSO Alzheimer's, Stroke *&* 29 Other Neurological Disorders Sourcebook, 1st Edition

■

Breast Cancer Sourcebook

Basic Consumer Health Information about Breast Cancer, Including Diagnostic Methods, Treatment Options, Alternative Therapies, Self-Help Information, Related Health Concerns, Statistical and Demographic Data, and Facts for Men with Breast Cancer

Along with Reports on Current Research Initiatives, a Glossary of Related Medical Terms, and a Directory of Sources for Further Help and Information

Edited by Edward J. Prucha and Karen Bellenir. 600 pages. 2001. 0-7808-0244-6. $78.

SEE ALSO Cancer Sourcebook for Women, 1st and 2nd Editions, Women's Health Concerns Sourcebook

■

Burns Sourcebook

Basic Consumer Health Information about Various Types of Burns and Scalds, Including Flame, Heat, Cold, Electrical, Chemical, and Sun Burns

Along with Information on Short-Term and Long-Term Treatments, Tissue Reconstruction, Plastic Surgery, Prevention Suggestions, and First Aid

Edited by Allan R. Cook. 604 pages. 1999. 0-7808-0204-7. $78.

"This key reference guide is an invaluable addition to all health care and public libraries in confronting this ongoing health issue."
—*American Reference Books Annual, 2000*

"This is an exceptional addition to the series and is highly recommended for all consumer health collections, hospital libraries, and academic medical centers." — *E-Streams, Mar '00*

"Recommended reference source."
—*Booklist, American Library Association, Dec '99*

SEE ALSO Skin Disorders Sourcebook

■

Cancer Sourcebook, 1st Edition

Basic Information on Cancer Types, Symptoms, Diagnostic Methods, and Treatments, Including Statistics on Cancer Occurrences Worldwide and the Risks Associated with Known Carcinogens and Activities

Edited by Frank E. Bair. 932 pages. 1990. 1-55888-888-8. $78.

Cited in *Reference Sources for Small and Medium-Sized Libraries*, American Library Association, 1999

"Written in nontechnical language. Useful for patients, their families, medical professionals, and librarians."
—*Guide to Reference Books, 1996*

"Designed with the non-medical professional in mind. Libraries and medical facilities interested in patient education should certainly consider adding the *Cancer Sourcebook* to their holdings. This compact collection of reliable information . . . is an invaluable tool for helping patients and patients' families and friends to take the first steps in coping with the many difficulties of cancer."
—*Medical Reference Services Quarterly, Winter '91*

"Specifically created for the nontechnical reader . . . an important resource for the general reader trying to understand the complexities of cancer."
—*American Reference Books Annual, 1991*

"This publication's nontechnical nature and very comprehensive format make it useful for both the general public and undergraduate students."
—*Choice, Association of College and Research Libraries, Oct '90*

■

New Cancer Sourcebook, 2nd Edition

Basic Information about Major Forms and Stages of Cancer, Featuring Facts about Primary and Secondary Tumors of the Respiratory, Nervous, Lymphatic, Circulatory, Skeletal, and Gastrointestinal Systems, and Specific Organs; Statistical and Demographic Data; Treatment Options; and Strategies for Coping

Edited by Allan R. Cook. 1,313 pages. 1996. 0-7808-0041-9. $78.

"An excellent resource for patients with newly diagnosed cancer and their families. The dialogue is simple, direct, and comprehensive. Highly recommended for patients and families to aid in their understanding of cancer and its treatment."
—*Booklist Health Sciences Supplement, American Library Association, Oct '97*

"The amount of factual and useful information is extensive. The writing is very clear, geared to general readers. Recommended for all levels."
— *Choice, Association of College and Research Libraries, Jan '97*

Cancer Sourcebook, 3rd Edition

Basic Consumer Health Information about Major Forms and Stages of Cancer, Featuring Facts about Primary and Secondary Tumors of the Respiratory, Nervous, Lymphatic, Circulatory, Skeletal, and Gastrointestinal Systems, and Specific Organs

Along with Statistical and Demographic Data, Treatment Options, Strategies for Coping, a Glossary, and a Directory of Sources for Additional Help and Information

Edited by Edward J. Prucha. 1,069 pages. 2000. 0-7808-0227-6. $78.

"Recommended reference source."
— *Booklist, American Library Association, Dec '00*

Cancer Sourcebook for Women, 1st Edition

Basic Information about Specific Forms of Cancer That Affect Women, Featuring Facts about Breast Cancer, Cervical Cancer, Ovarian Cancer, Cancer of the Uterus and Uterine Sarcoma, Cancer of the Vagina, and Cancer of the Vulva; Statistical and Demographic Data; Treatments, Self-Help Management Suggestions, and Current Research Initiatives

Edited by Allan R. Cook and Peter D. Dresser. 524 pages. 1996. 0-7808-0076-1. $78.

". . . written in easily understandable, non-technical language. Recommended for public libraries or hospital and academic libraries that collect patient education or consumer health materials."
— *Medical Reference Services Quarterly, Spring '97*

"Would be of value in a consumer health library. . . . written with the health care consumer in mind. Medical jargon is at a minimum, and medical terms are explained in clear, understandable sentences."
— *Bulletin of the Medical Library Association, Oct '96*

"The availability under one cover of all these pertinent publications, grouped under cohesive headings, makes this certainly a most useful sourcebook."
— *Choice, Association of College and Research Libraries, Jun '96*

"Presents a comprehensive knowledge base for general readers. Men and women both benefit from the gold mine of information nestled between the two covers of this book. Recommended."
— *Academic Library Book Review, Summer '96*

"This timely book is highly recommended for consumer health and patient education collections in all libraries."
— *Library Journal, Apr '96*

SEE ALSO Breast Cancer Sourcebook, Women's Health Concerns Sourcebook

Cancer Sourcebook for Women, 2nd Edition

Basic Consumer Health Information about Specific Forms of Cancer That Affect Women, Including Cervical Cancer, Ovarian Cancer, Endometrial Cancer, Uterine Sarcoma, Vaginal Cancer, Vulvar Cancer, and Gestational Trophoblastic Tumor; and Featuring Statistical Information, Facts about Tests and Treatments, a Glossary of Cancer Terms, and an Extensive List of Additional Resources

Edited by Edward J. Prucha and Karen Bellenir. 600 pages. 2001. 0-7808-0226-8. $78.

SEE ALSO Breast Cancer Sourcebook, Women's Health Concerns Sourcebook

Cardiovascular Diseases & Disorders Sourcebook, 1st Edition

Basic Information about Cardiovascular Diseases and Disorders, Featuring Facts about the Cardiovascular System, Demographic and Statistical Data, Descriptions of Pharmacological and Surgical Interventions, Lifestyle Modifications, and a Special Section Focusing on Heart Disorders in Children

Edited by Karen Bellenir and Peter D. Dresser. 683 pages. 1995. 0-7808-0032-X. $78.

". . . comprehensive format provides an extensive overview on this subject."
— *Choice, Association of College and Research Libraries, Jun '96*

". . . an easily understood, complete, up-to-date resource. This well executed public health tool will make valuable information available to those that need it most, patients and their families. The typeface, sturdy non-reflective paper, and library binding add a feel of quality found wanting in other publications. Highly recommended for academic and general libraries. "
— *Academic Library Book Review, Summer '96*

SEE ALSO Healthy Heart Sourcebook for Women, Heart Diseases & Disorders Sourcebook, 2nd Edition

Caregiving Sourcebook

Basic Consumer Health Information for Caregivers, Including a Profile of Caregivers, Caregiving Responsibilities, Tips for Specific Conditions, Care Environments, and the Effects of Caregiving

Along with Legal Issues, Financial Concerns, Future Planning, a Glossary, and a Listing of Additional Resources

Edited by Joyce Brennfleck Shannon. 550 pages. 2001. 0-7808-0331-0. $78.

Colds, Flu & Other Common Ailments Sourcebook

Basic Consumer Health Information about Common Ailments and Injuries, Including Colds, Coughs, the Flu, Sinus Problems, Headaches, Fever, Nausea and Vomiting, Menstrual Cramps, Diarrhea, Constipation, Hemorrhoids, Back Pain, Dandruff, Dry and Itchy Skin, Cuts, Scrapes, Sprains, Bruises, and More

Along with Information about Prevention, Self-Care, Choosing a Doctor, Over-the-Counter Medications, Folk Remedies, and Alternative Therapies, and Including a Glossary of Important Terms and a Directory of Resources for Further Help and Information

Edited by Chad T. Kimball. 600 pages. 2001. 0-7808-0435-X. $78.

■

Communication Disorders Sourcebook

Basic Information about Deafness and Hearing Loss, Speech and Language Disorders, Voice Disorders, Balance and Vestibular Disorders, and Disorders of Smell, Taste, and Touch

Edited by Linda M. Ross. 533 pages. 1996. 0-7808-0077-X. $78.

"This is skillfully edited and is a welcome resource for the layperson. It should be found in every public and medical library." *— Booklist Health Sciences Supplement, American Library Association, Oct '97*

■

Congenital Disorders Sourcebook

Basic Information about Disorders Acquired during Gestation, Including Spina Bifida, Hydrocephalus, Cerebral Palsy, Heart Defects, Craniofacial Abnormalities, Fetal Alcohol Syndrome, and More

Along with Current Treatment Options and Statistical Data

Edited by Karen Bellenir. 607 pages. 1997. 0-7808-0205-5. $78.

"Recommended reference source."
— Booklist, American Library Association, Oct '97

SEE ALSO *Pregnancy & Birth Sourcebook*

■

Consumer Issues in Health Care Sourcebook

Basic Information about Health Care Fundamentals and Related Consumer Issues, Including Exams and Screening Tests, Physician Specialties, Choosing a Doctor, Using Prescription and Over-the-Counter Medications Safely, Avoiding Health Scams, Managing Common Health Risks in the Home, Care Options for Chronically or Terminally Ill Patients, and a List of Resources for Obtaining Help and Further Information

Edited by Karen Bellenir. 618 pages. 1998. 0-7808-0221-7. $78.

"Both public and academic libraries will want to have a copy in their collection for readers who are interested in self-education on health issues."
—American Reference Books Annual, 2000

"The editor has researched the literature from government agencies and others, saving readers the time and effort of having to do the research themselves. Recommended for public libraries."
— Reference and User Services Quarterly, American Library Association, Spring '99

"Recommended reference source."
— Booklist, American Library Association, Dec '98

■

Contagious & Non-Contagious Infectious Diseases Sourcebook

Basic Information about Contagious Diseases like Measles, Polio, Hepatitis B, and Infectious Mononucleosis, and Non-Contagious Infectious Diseases like Tetanus and Toxic Shock Syndrome, and Diseases Occurring as Secondary Infections Such as Shingles and Reye Syndrome

Along with Vaccination, Prevention, and Treatment Information, and a Section Describing Emerging Infectious Disease Threats

Edited by Karen Bellenir and Peter D. Dresser. 566 pages. 1996. 0-7808-0075-3. $78.

■

Death & Dying Sourcebook

Basic Consumer Health Information for the Layperson about End-of-Life Care and Related Ethical and Legal Issues, Including Chief Causes of Death, Autopsies, Pain Management for the Terminally Ill, Life Support Systems, Insurance, Euthanasia, Assisted Suicide, Hospice Programs, Living Wills, Funeral Planning, Counseling, Mourning, Organ Donation, and Physician Training

Along with Statistical Data, a Glossary, and Listings of Sources for Further Help and Information

Edited by Annemarie S. Muth. 641 pages. 1999. 0-7808-0230-6. $78.

"Recommended reference source."
—Booklist, American Library Association, Aug '00

"This book is a definite must for all those involved in end-of-life care." *— Doody's Review Service, 2000*

■

Diabetes Sourcebook, 1st Edition

Basic Information about Insulin-Dependent and Non-insulin-Dependent Diabetes Mellitus, Gestational Diabetes, and Diabetic Complications, Symptoms, Treatment, and Research Results, Including Statistics on Prevalence, Morbidity, and Mortality

Along with Source Listings for Further Help and Information

Edited by Karen Bellenir and Peter D. Dresser. 827 pages. 1994. 1-55888-751-2. $78.

"... very informative and understandable for the layperson without being simplistic. It provides a comprehensive overview for laypersons who want a general understanding of the disease or who want to focus on various aspects of the disease."
— *Bulletin of the Medical Library Association, Jan '96*

Diabetes Sourcebook, 2nd Edition

Basic Consumer Health Information about Type 1 Diabetes (Insulin-Dependent or Juvenile-Onset Diabetes), Type 2 (Noninsulin-Dependent or Adult-Onset Diabetes), Gestational Diabetes, and Related Disorders, Including Diabetes Prevalence Data, Management Issues, the Role of Diet and Exercise in Controlling Diabetes, Insulin and Other Diabetes Medicines, and Complications of Diabetes Such as Eye Diseases, Periodontal Disease, Amputation, and End-Stage Renal Disease

Along with Reports on Current Research Initiatives, a Glossary, and Resource Listings for Further Help and Information

Edited by Karen Bellenir. 688 pages. 1998. 0-7808-0224-1. $78.

"This comprehensive book is an excellent addition for high school, academic, medical, and public libraries. This volume is highly recommended."
— *American Reference Books Annual, 2000*

"An invaluable reference." — *Library Journal, May '00*

Selected as one of the 250 "Best Health Sciences Books of 1999." — *Doody's Rating Service, Mar-Apr 2000*

"Recommended reference source."
— *Booklist, American Library Association, Feb '99*

"... provides reliable mainstream medical information ... belongs on the shelves of any library with a consumer health collection." — *E-Streams, Sep '99*

"Provides useful information for the general public."
— *Healthlines, University of Michigan Health Management Research Center, Sep/Oct '99*

Diet & Nutrition Sourcebook, 1st Edition

Basic Information about Nutrition, Including the Dietary Guidelines for Americans, the Food Guide Pyramid, and Their Applications in Daily Diet, Nutritional Advice for Specific Age Groups, Current Nutritional Issues and Controversies, the New Food Label and How to Use It to Promote Healthy Eating, and Recent Developments in Nutritional Research

Edited by Dan R. Harris. 662 pages. 1996. 0-7808-0084-2. $78.

"Useful reference as a food and nutrition sourcebook for the general consumer." — *Booklist Health Sciences Supplement, American Library Association, Oct '97*

"Recommended for public libraries and medical libraries that receive general information requests on nutrition. It is readable and will appeal to those interested in learning more about healthy dietary practices."
— *Medical Reference Services Quarterly, Fall '97*

"An abundance of medical and social statistics is translated into readable information geared toward the general reader." — *Bookwatch, Mar '97*

"With dozens of questionable diet books on the market, it is so refreshing to find a reliable and factual reference book. Recommended to aspiring professionals, librarians, and others seeking and giving reliable dietary advice. An excellent compilation." — *Choice, Association of College and Research Libraries, Feb '97*

SEE ALSO *Digestive Diseases & Disorders Sourcebook, Gastrointestinal Diseases & Disorders Sourcebook*

Diet & Nutrition Sourcebook, 2nd Edition

Basic Consumer Health Information about Dietary Guidelines, Recommended Daily Intake Values, Vitamins, Minerals, Fiber, Fat, Weight Control, Dietary Supplements, and Food Additives

Along with Special Sections on Nutrition Needs throughout Life and Nutrition for People with Such Specific Medical Concerns as Allergies, High Blood Cholesterol, Hypertension, Diabetes, Celiac Disease, Seizure Disorders, Phenylketonuria (PKU), Cancer, and Eating Disorders, and Including Reports on Current Nutrition Research and Source Listings for Additional Help and Information

Edited by Karen Bellenir. 650 pages. 1999. 0-7808-0228-4. $78.

"This book is an excellent source of basic diet and nutrition information." — *Booklist Health Sciences Supplement, American Library Association, Dec '00*

"This reference document should be in any public library, but it would be a very good guide for beginning students in the health sciences. If the other books in this publisher's series are as good as this, they should all be in the health sciences collections."
— *American Reference Books Annual, 2000*

"This book is an excellent general nutrition reference for consumers who desire to take an active role in their health care for prevention. Consumers of all ages who select this book can feel confident they are receiving current and accurate information."
— *Journal of Nutrition for the Elderly, Vol. 19, No. 4, '00*

"Recommended reference source."
— *Booklist, American Library Association, Dec '99*

SEE ALSO *Digestive Diseases & Disorders Sourcebook, Gastrointestinal Diseases & Disorders Sourcebook*

Digestive Diseases & Disorders Sourcebook

Basic Consumer Health Information about Diseases and Disorders that Impact the Upper and Lower Digestive System, Including Celiac Disease, Constipation, Crohn's Disease, Cyclic Vomiting Syndrome, Diarrhea, Diverticulosis and Diverticulitis, Gallstones, Heart-

burn, Hemorrhoids, Hernias, Indigestion (Dyspepsia), Irritable Bowel Syndrome, Lactose Intolerance, Ulcers, and More

Along with Information about Medications and Other Treatments, Tips for Maintaining a Healthy Digestive Tract, a Glossary, and Directory of Digestive Diseases Organizations

Edited by Karen Bellenir. 335 pages. 1999. 0-7808-0327-2. $48.

"This title is recommended for public, hospital, and health sciences libraries with consumer health collections." —*E-Streams, Jul-Aug '00*

"Recommended reference source."
—*Booklist, American Library Association, May '00*

SEE ALSO *Diet & Nutrition Sourcebook, 1st and 2nd Editions, Gastrointestinal Diseases & Disorders Sourcebook*

Disabilities Sourcebook

Basic Consumer Health Information about Physical and Psychiatric Disabilities, Including Descriptions of Major Causes of Disability, Assistive and Adaptive Aids, Workplace Issues, and Accessibility Concerns

Along with Information about the Americans with Disabilities Act, a Glossary, and Resources for Additional Help and Information

Edited by Dawn D. Matthews. 616 pages. 2000. 0-7808-0389-2. $78.

"An excellent source book in easy-to-read format covering many current topics; highly recommended for all libraries."
— *Choice, Association of College and Research Libraries, Jan '01*

"Recommended reference source."
—*Booklist, American Library Association, Jul '00*

"An involving, invaluable handbook."
—*The Bookwatch, May '00*

Domestic Violence & Child Abuse Sourcebook

Basic Consumer Health Information about Spousal/ Partner, Child, Sibling, Parent, and Elder Abuse, Covering Physical, Emotional, and Sexual Abuse, Teen Dating Violence, and Stalking; Includes Information about Hotlines, Safe Houses, Safety Plans, and Other Resources for Support and Assistance, Community Initiatives, and Reports on Current Directions in Research and Treatment

Along with a Glossary, Sources for Further Reading, and Governmental and Non-Governmental Organizations Contact Information

Edited by Helene Henderson. 1,064 pages. 2000. 0-7808-0235-7. $78.

Drug Abuse Sourcebook

Basic Consumer Health Information about Illicit Substances of Abuse and the Diversion of Prescription Medications, Including Depressants, Hallucinogens, Inhalants, Marijuana, Narcotics, Stimulants, and Anabolic Steroids

Along with Facts about Related Health Risks, Treatment Issues, and Substance Abuse Prevention Programs, a Glossary of Terms, Statistical Data, and Directories of Hotline Services, Self-Help Groups, and Organizations Able to Provide Further Information

Edited by Karen Bellenir. 629 pages. 2000. 0-7808-0242-X. $78.

"Highly recommended." — *The Bookwatch, Jan '01*

SEE ALSO *Alcoholism Sourcebook, Substance Abuse Sourcebook*

Ear, Nose & Throat Disorders Sourcebook

Basic Information about Disorders of the Ears, Nose, Sinus Cavities, Pharynx, and Larynx, Including Ear Infections, Tinnitus, Vestibular Disorders, Allergic and Non-Allergic Rhinitis, Sore Throats, Tonsillitis, and Cancers That Affect the Ears, Nose, Sinuses, and Throat

Along with Reports on Current Research Initiatives, a Glossary of Related Medical Terms, and a Directory of Sources for Further Help and Information

Edited by Karen Bellenir and Linda M. Shin. 576 pages. 1998. 0-7808-0206-3. $78.

"Overall, this sourcebook is helpful for the consumer seeking information on ENT issues. It is recommended for public libraries."
—*American Reference Books Annual, 1999*

"Recommended reference source."
—*Booklist, American Library Association, Dec '98*

Endocrine & Metabolic Disorders Sourcebook

Basic Information for the Layperson about Pancreatic and Insulin-Related Disorders Such as Pancreatitis, Diabetes, and Hypoglycemia; Adrenal Gland Disorders Such as Cushing's Syndrome, Addison's Disease, and Congenital Adrenal Hyperplasia; Pituitary Gland Disorders Such as Growth Hormone Deficiency, Acromegaly, and Pituitary Tumors; Thyroid Disorders Such as Hypothyroidism, Graves' Disease, Hashimoto's Disease, and Goiter; Hyperparathyroidism; and Other Diseases and Syndromes of Hormone Imbalance or Metabolic Dysfunction

Along with Reports on Current Research Initiatives

Edited by Linda M. Shin. 574 pages. 1998. 0-7808-0207-1. $78.

"Omnigraphics has produced another needed resource for health information consumers."
—*American Reference Books Annual, 2000*

"Recommended reference source."
— *Booklist, American Library Association, Dec '98*

Environmentally Induced Disorders Sourcebook

Basic Information about Diseases and Syndromes Linked to Exposure to Pollutants and Other Substances in Outdoor and Indoor Environments Such as Lead, Asbestos, Formaldehyde, Mercury, Emissions, Noise, and More

Edited by Allan R. Cook. 620 pages. 1997. 0-7808-0083-4. $78.

"Recommended reference source."
— *Booklist, American Library Association, Sep '98*

"This book will be a useful addition to anyone's library." — *Choice Health Sciences Supplement, Association of College and Research Libraries, May '98*

". . . a good survey of numerous environmentally induced physical disorders . . . a useful addition to anyone's library."
— *Doody's Health Sciences Book Reviews, Jan '98*

". . . provide[s] introductory information from the best authorities around. Since this volume covers topics that potentially affect everyone, it will surely be one of the most frequently consulted volumes in the *Health Reference Series*." — *Rettig on Reference, Nov '97*

Ethnic Diseases Sourcebook

Basic Consumer Health Information for Ethnic and Racial Minority Groups in the United States, Including General Health Indicators and Behaviors, Ethnic Diseases, Genetic Testing, the Impact of Chronic Diseases, Women's Health, Mental Health Issues, and Preventive Health Care Services

Along with a Glossary and a Listing of Additional Resources

Edited by Joyce Brennfleck Shannon. 600 pages. 2001. 0-7808-0336-1. $78.

Family Planning Sourcebook

Basic Consumer Health Information about Planning for Pregnancy and Contraception, Including Traditional Methods, Barrier Methods, Hormonal Methods, Permanent Methods, Future Methods, Emergency Contraception, and Birth Control Choices for Women at Each Stage of Life

Along with Statistics, a Glossary, and Sources of Additional Information

Edited by Amy Marcaccio Keyzer. 600 pages. 2001. 0-7808-0379-5. $78.

SEE ALSO *Pregnancy & Birth Sourcebook*

Fitness & Exercise Sourcebook, 1st Edition

Basic Information on Fitness and Exercise, Including Fitness Activities for Specific Age Groups, Exercise for People with Specific Medical Conditions, How to Begin a Fitness Program in Running, Walking, Swimming, Cycling, and Other Athletic Activities, and Recent Research in Fitness and Exercise

Edited by Dan R. Harris. 663 pages. 1996. 0-7808-0186-5. $78.

"A good resource for general readers."
— *Choice, Association of College and Research Libraries, Nov '97*

"The perennial popularity of the topic . . . make this an appealing selection for public libraries."
— *Rettig on Reference, Jun/Jul '97*

Fitness & Exercise Sourcebook, 2nd Edition

Basic Consumer Health Information about the Fundamentals of Fitness and Exercise, Including How to Begin and Maintain a Fitness Program, Fitness as a Lifestyle, the Link between Fitness and Diet, Advice for Specific Groups of People, Exercise as It Relates to Specific Medical Conditions, and Recent Research in Fitness and Exercise

Along with a Glossary of Important Terms and Resources for Additional Help and Information

Edited by Kristen M. Gledhill. 600 pages. 2001. 0-7808-0334-5. $78.

Food & Animal Borne Diseases Sourcebook

Basic Information about Diseases That Can Be Spread to Humans through the Ingestion of Contaminated Food or Water or by Contact with Infected Animals and Insects, Such as Botulism, E. Coli, Hepatitis A, Trichinosis, Lyme Disease, and Rabies

Along with Information Regarding Prevention and Treatment Methods, and Including a Special Section for International Travelers Describing Diseases Such as Cholera, Malaria, Travelers' Diarrhea, and Yellow Fever, and Offering Recommendations for Avoiding Illness

Edited by Karen Bellenir and Peter D. Dresser. 535 pages. 1995. 0-7808-0033-8. $78.

"Targeting general readers and providing them with a single, comprehensive source of information on selected topics, this book continues, with the excellent caliber of its predecessors, to catalog topical information on health matters of general interest. Readable and thorough, this valuable resource is highly recommended for all libraries."
— *Academic Library Book Review, Summer '96*

"A comprehensive collection of authoritative information." — *Emergency Medical Services, Oct '95*

Food Safety Sourcebook

Basic Consumer Health Information about the Safe Handling of Meat, Poultry, Seafood, Eggs, Fruit Juices, and Other Food Items, and Facts about Pesticides, Drinking Water, Food Safety Overseas, and the Onset, Duration, and Symptoms of Foodborne Illnesses, Including Types of Pathogenic Bacteria, Parasitic Protozoa, Worms, Viruses, and Natural Toxins

Along with the Role of the Consumer, the Food Handler, and the Government in Food Safety; a Glossary, and Resources for Additional Help and Information

Edited by Dawn D. Matthews. 339 pages. 1999. 0-7808-0326-4. $48.

"This book is recommended for public libraries and universities with home economic and food science programs." — *E-Streams, Nov '00*

"This book takes the complex issues of food safety and foodborne pathogens and presents them in an easily understood manner. [It does] an excellent job of covering a large and often confusing topic."
— *American Reference Books Annual, 2000*

"Recommended reference source."
— *Booklist, American Library Association, May '00*

Forensic Medicine Sourcebook

Basic Consumer Information for the Layperson about Forensic Medicine, Including Crime Scene Investigation, Evidence Collection and Analysis, Expert Testimony, Computer-Aided Criminal Identification, Digital Imaging in the Courtroom, DNA Profiling, Accident Reconstruction, Autopsies, Ballistics, Drugs and Explosives Detection, Latent Fingerprints, Product Tampering, and Questioned Document Examination

Along with Statistical Data, a Glossary of Forensics Terminology, and Listings of Sources for Further Help and Information

Edited by Annemarie S. Muth. 574 pages. 1999. 0-7808-0232-2. $78.

"There are several items that make this book attractive to consumers who are seeking certain forensic data. . . . This is a useful current source for those seeking general forensic medical answers."
— *American Reference Books Annual, 2000*

"Recommended for public libraries."
— *Reference & User Services Quarterly, American Library Association, Spring 2000*

"Recommended reference source."
— *Booklist, American Library Association, Feb '00*

"A wealth of information, useful statistics, references are up-to-date and extremely complete. This wonderful collection of data will help students who are interested in a career in any type of forensic field. It is a great resource for attorneys who need information about types of expert witnesses needed in a particular case. It also offers useful information for fiction and nonfiction writers whose work involves a crime. A fascinating compilation. All levels." — *Choice, Association of College and Research Libraries, Jan 2000*

Gastrointestinal Diseases & Disorders Sourcebook

Basic Information about Gastroesophageal Reflux Disease (Heartburn), Ulcers, Diverticulosis, Irritable Bowel Syndrome, Crohn's Disease, Ulcerative Colitis, Diarrhea, Constipation, Lactose Intolerance, Hemorrhoids, Hepatitis, Cirrhosis, and Other Digestive Problems, Featuring Statistics, Descriptions of Symptoms, and Current Treatment Methods of Interest for Persons Living with Upper and Lower Gastrointestinal Maladies

Edited by Linda M. Ross. 413 pages. 1996. 0-7808-0078-8. $78.

". . . very readable form. The successful editorial work that brought this material together into a useful and understandable reference makes accessible to all readers information that can help them more effectively understand and obtain help for digestive tract problems."
— *Choice, Association of College and Research Libraries, Feb '97*

SEE ALSO Diet & Nutrition Sourcebook, 1st and 2nd Editions, Digestive Diseases & Disorders Sourcebook

Genetic Disorders Sourcebook, 1st Edition

Basic Information about Heritable Diseases and Disorders Such as Down Syndrome, PKU, Hemophilia, Von Willebrand Disease, Gaucher Disease, Tay-Sachs Disease, and Sickle-Cell Disease, Along with Information about Genetic Screening, Gene Therapy, Home Care, and Including Source Listings for Further Help and Information on More Than 300 Disorders

Edited by Karen Bellenir. 642 pages. 1996. 0-7808-0034-6. $78.

"Recommended for undergraduate libraries or libraries that serve the public."
— *Science & Technology Libraries, Vol. 18, No. 1, '99*

"Provides essential medical information to both the general public and those diagnosed with a serious or fatal genetic disease or disorder."
— *Choice, Association of College and Research Libraries, Jan '97*

"Geared toward the lay public. It would be well placed in all public libraries and in those hospital and medical libraries in which access to genetic references is limited." — *Doody's Health Sciences Book Review, Oct '96*

Genetic Disorders Sourcebook, 2nd Edition

Basic Consumer Health Information about Hereditary Diseases and Disorders, Including Cystic Fibrosis, Down Syndrome, Hemophilia, Huntington's Disease, Sickle Cell Anemia, and More; Facts about Genes, Gene Research and Therapy, Genetic Screening, Ethics of Gene Testing, Genetic Counseling, and Advice on Coping and Caring

Along with a Glossary of Genetic Terminology and a Resource List for Help, Support, and Further Information

Edited by Kathy Massimini. 768 pages. 2001. 0-7808-0241-1. $78.

■

Head Trauma Sourcebook

Basic Information for the Layperson about Open-Head and Closed-Head Injuries, Treatment Advances, Recovery, and Rehabilitation

Along with Reports on Current Research Initiatives

Edited by Karen Bellenir. 414 pages. 1997. 0-7808-0208-X. $78.

■

Health Insurance Sourcebook

Basic Information about Managed Care Organizations, Traditional Fee-for-Service Insurance, Insurance Portability and Pre-Existing Conditions Clauses, Medicare, Medicaid, Social Security, and Military Health Care

Along with Information about Insurance Fraud

Edited by Wendy Wilcox. 530 pages. 1997. 0-7808-0222-5. $78.

"Particularly useful because it brings much of this information together in one volume. This book will be a handy reference source in the health sciences library, hospital library, college and university library, and medium to large public library."
—*Medical Reference Services Quarterly, Fall '98*

Awarded "Books of the Year Award"
—*American Journal of Nursing, 1997*

"The layout of the book is particularly helpful as it provides easy access to reference material. A most useful addition to the vast amount of information about health insurance. The use of data from U.S. government agencies is most commendable. Useful in a library or learning center for healthcare professional students."
—*Doody's Health Sciences Book Reviews, Nov '97*

■

Healthy Aging Sourcebook

Basic Consumer Health Information about Maintaining Health through the Aging Process, Including Advice on Nutrition, Exercise, and Sleep, Help in Making Decisions about Midlife Issues and Retirement, and Guidance Concerning Practical and Informed Choices in Health Consumerism

Along with Data Concerning the Theories of Aging, Different Experiences in Aging by Minority Groups, and Facts about Aging Now and Aging in the Future; and Featuring a Glossary, a Guide to Consumer Help, Additional Suggested Reading, and Practical Resource Directory

Edited by Jenifer Swanson. 536 pages. 1999. 0-7808-0390-6. $78.

"Recommended reference source."
—*Booklist, American Library Association, Feb '00*

SEE ALSO Physical & Mental Issues in Aging Sourcebook

Healthy Heart Sourcebook for Women

Basic Consumer Health Information about Cardiac Issues Specific to Women, Including Facts about Major Risk Factors and Prevention, Treatment and Control Strategies, and Important Dietary Issues

Along with a Special Section Regarding the Pros and Cons of Hormone Replacement Therapy and Its Impact on Heart Health, and Additional Help, Including Recipes, a Glossary, and a Directory of Resources

Edited by Dawn D. Matthews. 336 pages. 2000. 0-7808-0329-9. $48.

"Contains very important information about coronary artery disease that all women should know. The information is current and presented in an easy-to-read format. The book will make a good addition to any library."
—*American Medical Writers Association Journal, Summer '00*

"Important, basic reference."
—*Reviewer's Bookwatch, Jul '00*

SEE ALSO Cardiovascular Diseases & Disorders Sourcebook, 1st Edition, Heart Diseases & Disorders Sourcebook, 2nd Edition, Women's Health Concerns Sourcebook

■

Heart Diseases & Disorders Sourcebook, 2nd Edition

Basic Consumer Health Information about Heart Attacks, Angina, Rhythm Disorders, Heart Failure, Valve Disease, Congenital Heart Disorders, and More, Including Descriptions of Surgical Procedures and Other Interventions, Medications, Cardiac Rehabilitation, Risk Identification, and Prevention Tips

Along with Statistical Data, Reports on Current Research Initiatives, a Glossary of Cardiovascular Terms, and Resource Directory

Edited by Karen Bellenir. 612 pages. 2000. 0-7808-0238-1. $78.

"Recommended reference source."
—*Booklist, American Library Association, Dec '00*

"Provides comprehensive coverage of matters related to the heart. This title is recommended for health sciences and public libraries with consumer health collections."
—*E-Streams, Oct '00*

SEE ALSO Cardiovascular Diseases & Disorders Sourcebook, 1st Edition, Healthy Heart Sourcebook for Women

■

Immune System Disorders Sourcebook

Basic Information about Lupus, Multiple Sclerosis, Guillain-Barré Syndrome, Chronic Granulomatous Disease, and More

Along with Statistical and Demographic Data and Reports on Current Research Initiatives

Edited by Allan R. Cook. 608 pages. 1997. 0-7808-0209-8. $78.

Infant & Toddler Health Sourcebook

Basic Consumer Health Information about the Physical and Mental Development of Newborns, Infants, and Toddlers, Including Neonatal Concerns, Nutrition Recommendations, Immunization Schedules, Common Pediatric Disorders, Assessments and Milestones, Safety Tips, and Advice for Parents and Other Caregivers

Along with a Glossary of Terms and Resource Listings for Additional Help

Edited by Jenifer Swanson. 585 pages. 2000. 0-7808-0246-2. $78.

Kidney & Urinary Tract Diseases & Disorders Sourcebook

Basic Information about Kidney Stones, Urinary Incontinence, Bladder Disease, End Stage Renal Disease, Dialysis, and More

Along with Statistical and Demographic Data and Reports on Current Research Initiatives

Edited by Linda M. Ross. 602 pages. 1997. 0-7808-0079-6. $78.

Learning Disabilities Sourcebook

Basic Information about Disorders Such as Dyslexia, Visual and Auditory Processing Deficits, Attention Deficit/Hyperactivity Disorder, and Autism

Along with Statistical and Demographic Data, Reports on Current Research Initiatives, an Explanation of the Assessment Process, and a Special Section for Adults with Learning Disabilities

Edited by Linda M. Shin. 579 pages. 1998. 0-7808-0210-1. $78.

Named "Outstanding Reference Book of 1999."
— New York Public Library, Feb 2000

"An excellent candidate for inclusion in a public library reference section. It's a great source of information. Teachers will also find the book useful. Definitely worth reading."
— Journal of Adolescent & Adult Literacy, Feb 2000

"Readable . . . provides a solid base of information regarding successful techniques used with individuals who have learning disabilities, as well as practical suggestions for educators and family members. Clear language, concise descriptions, and pertinent information for contacting multiple resources add to the strength of this book as a useful tool."
— Choice, Association of College and Research Libraries, Feb '99

"Recommended reference source."
— Booklist, American Library Association, Sep '98

"This is a useful resource for libraries and for those who don't have the time to identify and locate the individual publications."
— Disability Resources Monthly, Sep '98

Liver Disorders Sourcebook

Basic Consumer Health Information about the Liver and How It Works; Liver Diseases, Including Cancer, Cirrhosis, Hepatitis, and Toxic and Drug Related Diseases; Tips for Maintaining a Healthy Liver; Laboratory Tests, Radiology Tests, and Facts about Liver Transplantation

Along with a Section on Support Groups, a Glossary, and Resource Listings

Edited by Joyce Brennfleck Shannon. 591 pages. 2000. 0-7808-0383-3. $78.

"This title is recommended for health sciences and public libraries with consumer health collections."
— E-Streams, Oct '00

"Recommended reference source."
— Booklist, American Library Association, Jun '00

Medical Tests Sourcebook

Basic Consumer Health Information about Medical Tests, Including Periodic Health Exams, General Screening Tests, Tests You Can Do at Home, Findings of the U.S. Preventive Services Task Force, X-ray and Radiology Tests, Electrical Tests, Tests of Blood and Other Body Fluids and Tissues, Scope Tests, Lung Tests, Genetic Tests, Pregnancy Tests, Newborn Screening Tests, Sexually Transmitted Disease Tests, and Computer Aided Diagnoses

Along with a Section on Paying for Medical Tests, a Glossary, and Resource Listings

Edited by Joyce Brennfleck Shannon. 691 pages. 1999. 0-7808-0243-8. $78.

"A valuable reference guide."
— American Reference Books Annual, 2000

"Recommended for hospital and health sciences libraries with consumer health collections."
— E-Streams, Mar '00

"This is an overall excellent reference with a wealth of general knowledge that may aid those who are reluctant to get vital tests performed."
— Today's Librarian, Jan 2000

Men's Health Concerns Sourcebook

Basic Information about Health Issues That Affect Men, Featuring Facts about the Top Causes of Death in Men, Including Heart Disease, Stroke, Cancers, Prostate Disorders, Chronic Obstructive Pulmonary Disease, Pneumonia and Influenza, Human Immunodeficiency Virus and Acquired Immune Deficiency Syndrome, Diabetes Mellitus, Stress, Suicide, Accidents and Homicides; and Facts about Common Concerns for Men, Including Impotence, Contraception, Circumcision, Sleep Disorders, Snoring, Hair Loss, Diet, Nutrition, Exercise, Kidney and Urological Disorders, and Backaches

Edited by Allan R. Cook. 738 pages. 1998. 0-7808-0212-8. $78.

■

Mental Health Disorders Sourcebook, 1st Edition

Basic Information about Schizophrenia, Depression, Bipolar Disorder, Panic Disorder, Obsessive-Compulsive Disorder, Phobias and Other Anxiety Disorders, Paranoia and Other Personality Disorders, Eating Disorders, and Sleep Disorders

Along with Information about Treatment and Therapies

Edited by Karen Bellenir. 548 pages. 1995. 0-7808-0040-0. $78.

■

Mental Health Disorders Sourcebook, 2nd Edition

Basic Consumer Health Information about Anxiety Disorders, Depression and Other Mood Disorders, Eating Disorders, Personality Disorders, Schizophrenia, and More, Including Disease Descriptions, Treatment Options, and Reports on Current Research Initiatives

Along with Statistical Data, Tips for Maintaining Mental Health, a Glossary, and Directory of Sources for Additional Help and Information

Edited by Karen Bellenir. 605 pages. 2000. 0-7808-0240-3. $78.

Mental Retardation Sourcebook

Basic Consumer Health Information about Mental Retardation and Its Causes, Including Down Syndrome, Fetal Alcohol Syndrome, Fragile X Syndrome, Genetic Conditions, Injury, and Environmental Sources

Along with Preventive Strategies, Parenting Issues, Educational Implications, Health Care Needs, Employment and Economic Matters, Legal Issues, a Glossary, and a Resource Listing for Additional Help and Information

Edited by Joyce Brennfleck Shannon. 642 pages. 2000. 0-7808-0377-9. $78.

■

Obesity Sourcebook

Basic Consumer Health Information about Diseases and Other Problems Associated with Obesity, and Including Facts about Risk Factors, Prevention Issues, and Management Approaches

Along with Statistical and Demographic Data, Information about Special Populations, Research Updates, a Glossary, and Source Listings for Further Help and Information

Edited by Wilma Caldwell and Chad T. Kimball. 376 pages. 2001. 0-7808-0333-7. $48.

■

Ophthalmic Disorders Sourcebook

Basic Information about Glaucoma, Cataracts, Macular Degeneration, Strabismus, Refractive Disorders, and More

Along with Statistical and Demographic Data and Reports on Current Research Initiatives

Edited by Linda M. Ross. 631 pages. 1996. 0-7808-0081-8. $78.

■

Oral Health Sourcebook

Basic Information about Diseases and Conditions Affecting Oral Health, Including Cavities, Gum Disease, Dry Mouth, Oral Cancers, Fever Blisters, Canker Sores, Oral Thrush, Bad Breath, Temporomandibular Disorders, and other Craniofacial Syndromes

Along with Statistical Data on the Oral Health of Americans, Oral Hygiene, Emergency First Aid, Information on Treatment Procedures and Methods of Replacing Lost Teeth

Edited by Allan R. Cook. 558 pages. 1997. 0-7808-0082-6. $78.

"Unique source which will fill a gap in dental sources for patients and the lay public. A valuable reference tool even in a library with thousands of books on dentistry. Comprehensive, clear, inexpensive, and easy to read and use. It fills an enormous gap in the health care literature."
— *Reference and User Services Quarterly, American Library Association, Summer '98*

"Recommended reference source."
— *Booklist, American Library Association, Dec '97*

■

Osteoporosis Sourcebook

Basic Consumer Health Information about Primary and Secondary Osteoporosis and Juvenile Osteoporosis and Related Conditions, Including Fibrous Dysplasia, Gaucher Disease, Hyperthyroidism, Hypophosphatasia, Myeloma, Osteopetrosis, Osteogenesis Imperfecta, and Paget's Disease

Along with Information about Risk Factors, Treatments, Traditional and Non-traditional Pain Management, a Glossary of Related Terms, and a Directory of Resources

Edited by Allan R. Cook. 600 pages. 2001. 0-7808-0239-X. $78.

SEE ALSO Women's Health Concerns Sourcebook

■

Pain Sourcebook

Basic Information about Specific Forms of Acute and Chronic Pain, Including Headaches, Back Pain, Muscular Pain, Neuralgia, Surgical Pain, and Cancer Pain

Along with Pain Relief Options Such as Analgesics, Narcotics, Nerve Blocks, Transcutaneous Nerve Stimulation, and Alternative Forms of Pain Control, Including Biofeedback, Imaging, Behavior Modification, and Relaxation Techniques

Edited by Allan R. Cook. 667 pages. 1997. 0-7808-0213-6. $78.

"The text is readable, easily understood, and well indexed. This excellent volume belongs in all patient education libraries, consumer health sections of public libraries, and many personal collections."
— *American Reference Books Annual, 1999*

"A beneficial reference." — *Booklist Health Sciences Supplement, American Library Association, Oct '98*

"The information is basic in terms of scholarship and is appropriate for general readers. Written in journalistic style . . . intended for non-professionals. Quite thorough in its coverage of different pain conditions and summarizes the latest clinical information regarding pain treatment." — *Choice, Association of College and Research Libraries, Jun '98*

"Recommended reference source."
— *Booklist, American Library Association, Mar '98*

Pediatric Cancer Sourcebook

Basic Consumer Health Information about Leukemias, Brain Tumors, Sarcomas, Lymphomas, and Other Cancers in Infants, Children, and Adolescents, Including Descriptions of Cancers, Treatments, and Coping Strategies

Along with Suggestions for Parents, Caregivers, and Concerned Relatives, a Glossary of Cancer Terms, and Resource Listings

Edited by Edward J. Prucha. 587 pages. 1999. 0-7808-0245-4. $78.

"A valuable addition to all libraries specializing in health services and many public libraries."
— *American Reference Books Annual, 2000*

"Recommended reference source."
— *Booklist, American Library Association, Feb '00*

"An excellent source of information. Recommended for public, hospital, and health science libraries with consumer health collections." — *E-Streams, Jun '00*

■

Physical & Mental Issues in Aging Sourcebook

Basic Consumer Health Information on Physical and Mental Disorders Associated with the Aging Process, Including Concerns about Cardiovascular Disease, Pulmonary Disease, Oral Health, Digestive Disorders, Musculoskeletal and Skin Disorders, Metabolic Changes, Sexual and Reproductive Issues, and Changes in Vision, Hearing, and Other Senses

Along with Data about Longevity and Causes of Death, Information on Acute and Chronic Pain, Descriptions of Mental Concerns, a Glossary of Terms, and Resource Listings for Additional Help

Edited by Jenifer Swanson. 660 pages. 1999. 0-7808-0233-0. $78.

"Recommended for public libraries."
— *American Reference Books Annual, 2000*

"This is a treasure of health information for the layperson." — *Choice Health Sciences Supplement, Association of College & Research Libraries, May 2000*

"Recommended reference source."
— *Booklist, American Library Association, Oct '99*

SEE ALSO Healthy Aging Sourcebook

■

Podiatry Sourcebook

Basic Consumer Health Information about Foot Conditions, Diseases, and Injuries, Including Bunions, Corns, Calluses, Athlete's Foot, Plantar Warts, Hammertoes and Clawtoes, Club Foot, Heel Pain, Gout, and More

Along with Facts about Foot Care, Disease Prevention, Foot Safety, Choosing a Foot Care Specialist, a Glossary of Terms, and Resource Listings for Additional Information

Edited by M. Lisa Weatherford. 600 pages. 2001. 0-7808-0215-2. $78.

Pregnancy & Birth Sourcebook

Basic Information about Planning for Pregnancy, Maternal Health, Fetal Growth and Development, Labor and Delivery, Postpartum and Perinatal Care, Pregnancy in Mothers with Special Concerns, and Disorders of Pregnancy, Including Genetic Counseling, Nutrition and Exercise, Obstetrical Tests, Pregnancy Discomfort, Multiple Births, Cesarean Sections, Medical Testing of Newborns, Breastfeeding, Gestational Diabetes, and Ectopic Pregnancy

Edited by Heather E. Aldred. 737 pages. 1997. 0-7808-0216-0. $78.

"A well-organized handbook. Recommended."
— *Choice, Association of College and Research Libraries, Apr '98*

"Recommended reference source."
— *Booklist, American Library Association, Mar '98*

"Recommended for public libraries."
— *American Reference Books Annual, 1998*

SEE ALSO *Congenital Disorders Sourcebook, Family Planning Sourcebook*

Public Health Sourcebook

Basic Information about Government Health Agencies, Including National Health Statistics and Trends, Healthy People 2000 Program Goals and Objectives, the Centers for Disease Control and Prevention, the Food and Drug Administration, and the National Institutes of Health

Along with Full Contact Information for Each Agency

Edited by Wendy Wilcox. 698 pages. 1998. 0-7808-0220-9. $78.

"Recommended reference source."
— *Booklist, American Library Association, Sep '98*

"This consumer guide provides welcome assistance in navigating the maze of federal health agencies and their data on public health concerns."
— *SciTech Book News, Sep '98*

Reconstructive & Cosmetic Surgery Sourcebook

Basic Consumer Health Information on Cosmetic and Reconstructive Plastic Surgery, Including Statistical Information about Different Surgical Procedures, Things to Consider Prior to Surgery, Plastic Surgery Techniques and Tools, Emotional and Psychological Considerations, and Procedure-Specific Information

Along with a Glossary of Terms and a Listing of Resources for Additional Help and Information

Edited by M. Lisa Weatherford. 374 pages. 2001. 0-7808-0214-4. $48.

Rehabilitation Sourcebook

Basic Consumer Health Information about Rehabilitation for People Recovering from Heart Surgery, Spinal Cord Injury, Stroke, Orthopedic Impairments, Amputation, Pulmonary Impairments, Traumatic Injury, and More, Including Physical Therapy, Occupational Therapy, Speech/ Language Therapy, Massage Therapy, Dance Therapy, Art Therapy, and Recreational Therapy

Along with Information on Assistive and Adaptive Devices, a Glossary, and Resources for Additional Help and Information

Edited by Dawn D. Matthews. 531 pages. 1999. 0-7808-0236-5. $78.

"Recommended reference source."
— *Booklist, American Library Association, May '00*

Respiratory Diseases & Disorders Sourcebook

Basic Information about Respiratory Diseases and Disorders, Including Asthma, Cystic Fibrosis, Pneumonia, the Common Cold, Influenza, and Others, Featuring Facts about the Respiratory System, Statistical and Demographic Data, Treatments, Self-Help Management Suggestions, and Current Research Initiatives

Edited by Allan R. Cook and Peter D. Dresser. 771 pages. 1995. 0-7808-0037-0. $78.

"Designed for the layperson and for patients and their families coping with respiratory illness. . . . an extensive array of information on diagnosis, treatment, management, and prevention of respiratory illnesses for the general reader." — *Choice, Association of College and Research Libraries, Jun '96*

"A highly recommended text for all collections. It is a comforting reminder of the power of knowledge that good books carry between their covers."
— *Academic Library Book Review, Spring '96*

"A comprehensive collection of authoritative information presented in a nontechnical, humanitarian style for patients, families, and caregivers."
— *Association of Operating Room Nurses, Sep/Oct '95*

Sexually Transmitted Diseases Sourcebook, 1st Edition

Basic Information about Herpes, Chlamydia, Gonorrhea, Hepatitis, Nongonoccocal Urethritis, Pelvic Inflammatory Disease, Syphilis, AIDS, and More

Along with Current Data on Treatments and Preventions

Edited by Linda M. Ross. 550 pages. 1997. 0-7808-0217-9. $78.

Sexually Transmitted Diseases Sourcebook, 2nd Edition

Basic Consumer Health Information about Sexually Transmitted Diseases, Including Information on the Diagnosis and Treatment of Chlamydia, Gonorrhea, Hepatitis, Herpes, HIV, Mononucleosis, Syphilis, and Others

Along with Information on Prevention, Such as Condom Use, Vaccines, and STD Education; And Featuring a Section on Issues Related to Youth and Adolescents, a Glossary, and Resources for Additional Help and Information

Edited by Dawn D. Matthews. 538 pages. 2001. 0-7808-0249-7. $78.

■

Skin Disorders Sourcebook

Basic Information about Common Skin and Scalp Conditions Caused by Aging, Allergies, Immune Reactions, Sun Exposure, Infectious Organisms, Parasites, Cosmetics, and Skin Traumas, Including Abrasions, Cuts, and Pressure Sores

Along with Information on Prevention and Treatment

Edited by Allan R. Cook. 647 pages. 1997. 0-7808-0080-X. $78.

"... comprehensive, easily read reference book."
— *Doody's Health Sciences Book Reviews, Oct '97*

SEE ALSO *Burns Sourcebook*

■

Sleep Disorders Sourcebook

Basic Consumer Health Information about Sleep and Its Disorders, Including Insomnia, Sleepwalking, Sleep Apnea, Restless Leg Syndrome, and Narcolepsy

Along with Data about Shiftwork and Its Effects, Information on the Societal Costs of Sleep Deprivation, Descriptions of Treatment Options, a Glossary of Terms, and Resource Listings for Additional Help

Edited by Jenifer Swanson. 439 pages. 1998. 0-7808-0234-9. $78.

"This text will complement any home or medical library. It is user-friendly and ideal for the adult reader."
—*American Reference Books Annual, 2000*

"Recommended reference source."
— *Booklist, American Library Association, Feb '99*

"A useful resource that provides accurate, relevant, and accessible information on sleep to the general public. Health care providers who deal with sleep disorders patients may also find it helpful in being prepared to answer some of the questions patients ask."
—*Respiratory Care, Jul '99*

Sports Injuries Sourcebook

Basic Consumer Health Information about Common Sports Injuries, Prevention of Injury in Specific Sports, Tips for Training, and Rehabilitation from Injury

Along with Information about Special Concerns for Children, Young Girls in Athletic Training Programs, Senior Athletes, and Women Athletes, and a Directory of Resources for Further Help and Information

Edited by Heather E. Aldred. 624 pages. 1999. 0-7808-0218-7. $78.

"Public libraries and undergraduate academic libraries will find this book useful for its nontechnical language." —*American Reference Books Annual, 2000*

"While this easy-to-read book is recommended for all libraries, it should prove to be especially useful for public, high school, and academic libraries; certainly it should be on the bookshelf of every school gymnasium." —*E-Streams, Mar '00*

■

Substance Abuse Sourcebook

Basic Health-Related Information about the Abuse of Legal and Illegal Substances Such as Alcohol, Tobacco, Prescription Drugs, Marijuana, Cocaine, and Heroin; and Including Facts about Substance Abuse Prevention Strategies, Intervention Methods, Treatment and Recovery Programs, and a Section Addressing the Special Problems Related to Substance Abuse during Pregnancy

Edited by Karen Bellenir. 573 pages. 1996. 0-7808-0038-9. $78.

"A valuable addition to any health reference section. Highly recommended."
— *The Book Report, Mar/Apr '97*

"... a comprehensive collection of substance abuse information that's both highly readable and compact. Families and caregivers of substance abusers will find the information enlightening and helpful, while teachers, social workers and journalists should benefit from the concise format. Recommended."
— *Drug Abuse Update, Winter '96/'97*

SEE ALSO *Alcoholism Sourcebook, Drug Abuse Sourcebook*

■

Traveler's Health Sourcebook

Basic Consumer Health Information for Travelers, Including Physical and Medical Preparations, Transportation Health and Safety, Essential Information about Food and Water, Sun Exposure, Insect and Snake Bites, Camping and Wilderness Medicine, and Travel with Physical or Medical Disabilities

Along with International Travel Tips, Vaccination Recommendations, Geographical Health Issues, Disease Risks, a Glossary, and a Listing of Additional Resources

Edited by Joyce Brennfleck Shannon. 613 pages. 2000. 0-7808-0384-1. $78.

Women's Health Concerns Sourcebook

Basic Information about Health Issues That Affect Women, Featuring Facts about Menstruation and Other Gynecological Concerns, Including Endometriosis, Fibroids, Menopause, and Vaginitis; Reproductive Concerns, Including Birth Control, Infertility, and Abortion; and Facts about Additional Physical, Emotional, and Mental Health Concerns Prevalent among Women Such as Osteoporosis, Urinary Tract Disorders, Eating Disorders, and Depression

Along with Tips for Maintaining a Healthy Lifestyle

Edited by Heather E. Aldred. 567 pages. 1997. 0-7808-0219-5. $78.

"Handy compilation. There is an impressive range of diseases, devices, disorders, procedures, and other physical and emotional issues covered . . . well organized, illustrated, and indexed." — *Choice, Association of College and Research Libraries, Jan '98*

SEE ALSO *Breast Cancer Sourcebook, Cancer Sourcebook for Women, 1st and 2nd Editions, Healthy Heart Sourcebook for Women, Osteoporosis Sourcebook*

■

Workplace Health & Safety Sourcebook

Basic Consumer Health Information about Workplace Health and Safety, Including the Effect of Workplace Hazards on the Lungs, Skin, Heart, Ears, Eyes, Brain, Reproductive Organs, Musculoskeletal System, and Other Organs and Body Parts

Along with Information about Occupational Cancer, Personal Protective Equipment, Toxic and Hazardous Chemicals, Child Labor, Stress, and Workplace Violence

Edited by Chad T. Kimball. 626 pages. 2000. 0-7808-0231-4. $78.

"Highly recommended." — *The Bookwatch, Jan '01*

■

Worldwide Health Sourcebook

Basic Information about Global Health Issues, Including Malnutrition, Reproductive Health, Disease Dispersion and Prevention, Emerging Diseases, Risky Health Behaviors, and the Leading Causes of Death

Along with Global Health Concerns for Children, Women, and the Elderly, Mental Health Issues, Research and Technology Advancements, and Economic, Environmental, and Political Health Implications, a Glossary, and a Resource Listing for Additional Help and Information

Edited by Joyce Brennfleck Shannon. 500 pages. 2001. 0-7808-0330-2. $78.

Health Reference Series Cumulative Index 1999

A Comprehensive Index to the Individual Volumes of the Health Reference Series, Including a Subject Index, Name Index, Organization Index, and Publication Index

Along with a Master List of Acronyms and Abbreviations

Edited by Edward J. Prucha, Anne Holmes, and Robert Rudnick. 990 pages. 2000. 0-7808-0382-5. $78.

"Essential for collections that hold any of the numerous *Health Reference Series* titles." — *Choice, Association of College and Research Libraries, Nov '00*